New Directions in Old-Age Policies

New Directions
in Old-Age Policies

Janie S. Steckenrider
and Tonya M. Parrott

State University of New York Press

Published by
State University of New York Press, Albany

© 1998 State University of New York

For information, address State University of New York Press,
State University Plaza, Albany, N.Y. 12246

Production by Diane Ganeles
Marketing by Patrick Durocher

Library of Congress Cataloging-in-Publication Data

Steckenrider, Janie S., 1954–
    New directions in old-age policies / Janie S. Steckenrider and
Tonya M. Parrott.
        p. cm.
    Includes bibliographical references and index.
    ISBN 0-7914-3913-5 (hc : alk. paper). ISBN 0-7914-3914-3 (pbk.
: alk. paper)
    1. Old age—Government policy—United States. 2. Old age
assistance—Government policy—United States. 3. Aged—United
States—Social conditions. 4. Aged—United States—Economic
conditions. 5. United States—Social policy. 6. United States—
Politics and government. I. Parrott, Tonya M., 1968–
II. Title.
HQ1064.U5S699   1998
362.6'0973—dc21
                                                              97-46976
                                                                 CIP

10 9 8 7 6 5 4 3 2 1

Contents

List of Tables

List of Figures

Chapter 1

Introduction: The Political Environment and the New Face of Aging Policy

JANIE S. STECKENRIDER
AND TONYA M. PARROTT

Old-age policies in the United States are heading in new directions as the country enters the next millennium. Gone are the days of program growth, automatic increases, and expanded benefits for senior citizens. Aging policies, like other policy arenas, have changed (and been changed) in response to the fundamentally different political environment that swept the country during the late 1980s. The dominant themes of the current political environment are deficit reduction, program reform, state experimentation, elimination of waste and redundancy, and individual responsibility. These new themes coupled with the demographic forces of the growing number of elderly, especially as the Baby Boom ages toward retirement, have changed the face of aging policy. Aging policy encompasses the myriad of programs directed toward senior citizens and toward an aging population such as Medicare, Social Security, the Older Americans Act, home-delivered meals, subsidized housing, legal assistance, and transportation services.

Old-age policies and programs, constituting over one-third of the federal budget in the 1990s, face a new set of political priorities and constraints within the changed political landscape. Four related shifts loom large in guiding the aging policy responses to these changes: questioned legitimacy of the elderly as beneficiaries, decreased government responsibility offset by increased family responsibility, a bottom-line approach to all programs including those for seniors, and a dramatic change in political leadership in the mid-1990s. These changed perspectives underline how shifting values in the broader political spectrum impinge on specific policy arenas like aging.

Four Shifts Guiding Aging Policy

For many decades the elderly were presumed to be the most deserving of beneficiaries for government largess. They were often considered vulnerable and needy of services, economically hindered by fixed incomes, and respected for their lifetime of contributions to society. Large federal programs were government's answer for the elderly—Social Security and Supplemental Security Income for income maintenance and Medicare and Medicaid for health care; as well as programs of subsidized housing, energy assistance, transportation services, and legal aid. The budgets for age-related programs grew and the services provided continually expanded. The elderly were seen as such deserving program recipients that benefits were automatically expanded like the Cost of Living Adjustments for Social Security. This legitimacy of the elderly as beneficiaries is now under question. Increasingly seniors are called "Greedy Geezers," a pejorative term suggesting that the elderly are receiving too large a slice of the government pie. Claims for intergenerational equity have also made it into the public vernacular, emphasizing the need to distribute government benefits equally across the generations. Questioning whether the elderly may be "getting too much" of government's benefits—an idea unspeakable in earlier decades—is center stage in the present political environment.

By emphasizing the heterogeneity of the senior population, some of the criticisms about the elderly and the privileges they receive from the federal government have been made valid. For example, not all elderly are poor, alone, disabled, and living from one Social Security check to the next. The very success of many social programs for the elderly has added to the demise of the deserving status "the elderly" were given in earlier decades. It has become increasingly clear that "the elderly" as a group are less defendable as public program beneficiaries than are subgroups of the elderly most in need. Some consequences have been the targeting of services to subgroups, that is, poor, rural, and minority, and the increased assumption of such program costs by the elderly as raised Medicare Part B premiums.

The underlying values of public policy have also shifted as America enters the twenty-first century. The pendulum has swung toward decreased federal government responsibility in all areas. The burden is on states, cities, counties, the private sector, families, and individuals to bridge the gap and to assume more responsibility. Recent debates on welfare reform, Medicare cuts, and block grants reflect this devolving of the federal government. Aging policy, like the broader political environment, is being impacted by this shift in values toward individual responsibility. Monthly premiums for Medicare have been increased, Social Security benefits of the wealthier elderly have been taxed, the eligibility age for Social Security has been raised, social services for seniors have been increasingly targeted to low-income and minority elderly, and proposals for national long-term care insurance have been abandoned—all reflecting the underlying value in public policy that the individual, and for the elderly often their family, must assume a greater share of the responsibilities. Old-age policies have been impacted and altered by the decreased role of the federal government.

The third fundamental shift that pervades aging policy in the current political environment is the bottom-line cost approach with a near exclusive focus on what can be cut. The transition is one from earlier decades of program expansion to this new era of sustaining aging programs. Previously aging programs were considered the third rail of politics, "touch them and you die." But policymakers no longer view aging programs as sacred and untouchable. Every part of the federal budget, including aging programs, is under the budget-cutting microscope. And because old-age policies are so visible due to their immense size and costs, aging programs are now considered a central component of any budget proposal. The extent of this shift was symbolized by the debates of the 1996 federal budget that hinged entirely on the extent of cuts in the elderly health care program of Medicare. So intense was the political impasse of Congress and the president over balancing the budget and Medicare cuts that the federal government was shut down twice. Budget debates centering on how deep cuts should be in elderly programs are a far cry from the days of program expansion, legitimacy of benefits to seniors, and untouchable senior services.

Last, there was a dramatic change in the political leadership in the House and Senate from the 1994 midterm congressional elections, reversing forty years of Democratic leadership and accompanied by an intense focus on the House GOP Contract with America. This is important because the Republican agenda dominated the first hundred days; no other issues were given attention in Congress, including aging issues. Moreover, the shift from Democratic to Republican leadership in Congress meant that any chance of expanding health care benefits for the elderly or for any other group (so prominent a theme only two years earlier in the 1992 presidential campaign) were gone. Gone, too, was any possibility to develop long-term care options involving federal financing mechanisms (which seemed inevitable at the annual meeting of the Gerontological Society of America in 1994).

This change in leadership is crucial to a complete understanding of why aging programs were no longer given preferential treatment in Congress. Many aging advocates seemed caught off-guard by the ramifications of the leadership change and unclear where to focus their energies. The congressional leaders with whom many advocates had worked were no longer in power and there was no clear point-person to turn to for support (Liebig, 1995). Not only were aging policies given closer scrutiny in this new political environment, but aging advocates had to devise new strategies to work with the changed leaders, committees, and policy priorities.

It is not just the changed political environment that has impacted aging policies but other broad societal forces are coalescing to generate new directions in old-age policies. America is an increasingly aging nation—the population is getting older, people are living longer, there are more very old persons, and the enormous Baby Boom is quickly moving toward becoming a Senior Boom. (See Figure 1.1.) Plus, there are considerably more frail elderly as people are living longer once they reach old age. It is the frail elderly who are most in need of government services and those who are most costly. Aging policy in the twenty-first century has no choice but to adapt to these changing demographic characteristics.

Another significant societal trend is the cost of medical care that has mushroomed for all ages. The cost increases, however, are especially significant for the elderly since they are the biggest consumers of health care and the government provides their coverage through Medicare. Both Medicare and Social Security are projected to be bankrupt in the early decades of the twenty-first century that also is compelling changes in current aging policies to stall the demise of these programs. There is growing sentiment that changes to these programs need to be made now so that the Baby Boom generation receives, at the very least, something. Another force is

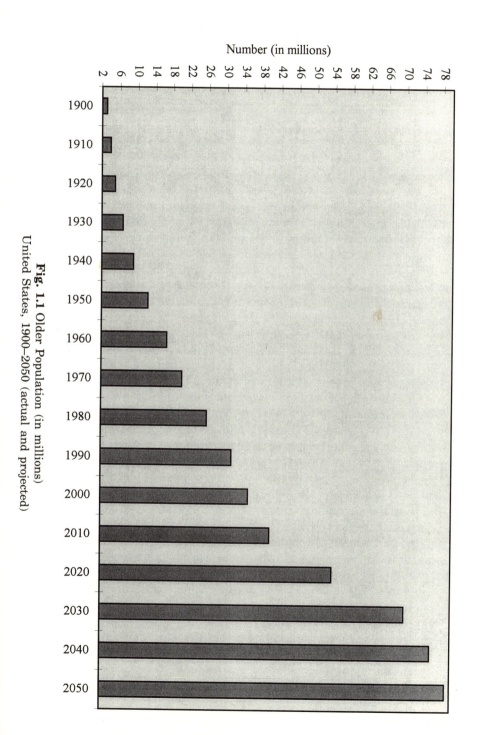

Fig. 1.1 Older Population (in millions)
United States, 1900–2050 (actual and projected)

the high cost of nursing home care that is crippling older persons and their families. Yet Medicaid, the only governmental support of long-term care, is continually facing state shortfalls in its funding. With the demographic trends ahead, the costs of long-term care are expected to increase significantly. These varied societal forces and the new concerns and priorities of the political environment mean that old-age policies must move in new directions.

New Directions in Old-Age Policies

As we enter the twenty-first century, researchers and advocates for the elderly are being forced to turn their critical lenses inward to question what has been achieved in old-age policy; what can be sustained in this current political environment; and what are the new directions, issues, and concerns for aging policy. *New Directions in Old Age Policies* explores two questions: (1) How is aging policy made within this current climate of budget restraints, deficits, cutbacks, program reductions, and legitimate competing interests? (2) What are the future prospects for old-age policies as the dramatic aging of the American population in the coming decades add future demands and pressures?

The policy solutions for issues of old age depend in part on the legislative and grass roots efforts of the 33.2 million persons over age 65, their advocates from organized interest groups (e.g., American Association of Retired Persons, National Senior Citizens Council, and Older Women's League), and on the public's perception of how needy the elderly are as a group compared to other deserving groups. But things have also changed for the elderly's advocates. The Senate hearings in 1995 on the tax-exempt status of the American Association for Retired Persons is evidence of the changes and that the Republican leadership was not afraid to take on the elderly and their advocates (Liebig, 1995). Today, maneuvering old-age policy through the policy system is far more difficult as the general focus on program cutbacks is accompanied by a questioning of the legitimacy of the elderly as recipients of government assistance. This changed political environment and the heightened questioning of legitimacy in turn calls on researchers to educate the public and policymakers on the realities of the elderly population, to identify and communicate the new issues in aging policy, and then to develop policy solutions that address these needs within the context of the new political environment.

The aging public policy literature presently has a gap in exploring the current and future issues within the different arenas of aging policy. To address this neglected area, this volume looks at the new directions in the specific policy arenas of (1) retirement policies and alternative financing mechanisms; (2) health care policies and reform; (3) housing policies and intergovernmental relationships; (4) interest group politics and strategies; (5) gender bias in aging policies and the plight of older women; (6) changing family demographics, caregiving demands, and policy needs; (7) the ethnic and racial diversity of the elderly facing policymakers; and (8) the competing claims of generational inequity. In each policy arena the possible solutions available to policymakers, given the current political environment, are explored.

While there are several books that address a single aging policy arena such as income maintenance, health care, housing, or older women, there are few books that bring together varying policy arenas into one volume and suggest the future direction of aging policy within the new political climate. Given the multiple policy areas that impact the lives of the elderly, this book provides a multipolicy perspective by addressing the new directions in aging policy in each of these arenas and draws together the policy solutions that take into account the reality of the new political landscape.

This volume is divided into three sections with each focusing on a different aspect of the impact of the changed political environment on aging policies. Section I, "Distinct Policy Domains: A Fresh Look at Old-Age Policies," focuses on three specific policy areas. Robert H. Binstock in "Health Care Policies and Older Americans" focuses on the issues shaping health care policies that affect older Americans. Reviewing the costs of health care and whether population aging has been a major factor in its growth, he also examines current efforts to curb Medicare and the dilemmas in financing long-term care. Different aspects of income maintenance policies are examined by Ying-Ping Chen as he considers Social Security and its current and future policy directions in "Economic Security: Strengthening Social Security and Private Pensions." Chen focuses on the underlying importance of Social Security for future generations of elderly and discusses the various options for shoring up the long-term stability of the system. The changes in housing policy are explored by Phoebe S. Liebig in "Housing and Supportive Services for the Elderly: Intragenerational Perspectives and Options" with an emphasis on intergovernmental relationships. She provides a housing profile of the elderly population and discusses various housing policies of the federal and state governments. Liebig explores the future of housing policy and suggests that housing inequality among the aged will persist because of forces within the new political environment.

Section II, "Politics and Aging Policy," focuses on the aspects of the political environment that have changed and that are prompting a new face to aging policies. Former assistant secretary for Aging, U.S. Department of Health and Human Services, Fernando M. Torres-Gil contributes an insider's view of policy-making for the elderly in "Policy, Politics, Aging: Crossroads in the 1990s." As the first head of the elevated Aging Department within the Department of Health and Human Services, Torres-Gil summarizes the history of aging policy and succinctly outlines the implications of the changed political environment for future aging policy. Another insider's view is provided by Robert B. Blancato, the chief organizer of the 1995 White Conference on Aging, and Brian W. Lindberg, a delegate in "The 1995 White House Conference on Aging: A Tradition Confronts a Revolution." Each White House Conference on Aging has led the way in setting the agenda for aging policy for the decade to come with early conferences laying the foundation for Medicare, Medicaid, the Older Americans Act, Supplemental Security Income, and Social Security amendments. Blancato and Lindberg discuss the process and the policy imperatives that developed from the 1995 conference and show how the changed political environment shaped the debates and issues.

Politically active and involved, senior citizens are believed by many to have capitalized on their clout in campaigns and elections to influence policymakers in policy debates. Susan MacManus and Kathryn Dunn Tenpas in "The Changing Political Activism Patterns of Older Americans: 'Don't Throw the Dirt Over Us Yet'" describe the current and future political participation of the senior population. Elderly interest groups have long been recognized as a powerful force in aging politics and a force to be reckoned with. However, elderly interest groups have experienced a changing role and increased challenges to their position. Based on interviews with interest group leaders and congressional staff members, Christine L. Day discusses the reaction of elderly interest groups to the new political forces and posits their future position in aging debates in "Old-Age Interest Groups in the 1990s: Coalitions, Competition, and Strategy."

Another major change in the political landscape has been the recent concerns with intergenerational equity and fairness across the generations in budgetary politics. Giving particular attention to spending preferences indicative of generational conflict over policy priorities, Laurie B. Rhodebeck examines public attitudes toward government spending and their relationship to congressional policy-making. In "Competing Problems, Budget Constraints, and Claims for Intergenerational Equity," Rhodebeck describes the development of the intergenerational equity issue and its role in recent budgetary politics affecting the elderly.

The diversity of the elderly population and the dilemmas posed by the specific subgroup populations is the theme for Section III, "The Family, Ethnicity, and Older Women: Aging Policy Dilemmas." As the federal government decreases its role and as more responsibilities are shifted to the individual, families are of critical importance to the elderly person for support and care. Tonya M. Parrott in "Changing Family Demographics, Caregiving Demands, and Policy Needs" discusses the intersection of family, policy, and an aging society within the context of the changing demographics of family life. She explores the future implications of these trends on help and support of older family members and identifies a diverse set of care arrangements that will require attention in future family policy decisions. Valentine M. Villa emphasizes the need to consider the ethnic diversity of the elderly population. In "The Status of Ethnic Minority Elderly: The Challenge to Policymakers," Villa provides an in-depth profile of the racial and ethnic composition of the elderly population. She demonstrates the critical need for policymakers to account for this diversity in aging policy and to be aware of the unintended consequences of broader policy changes on the elderly, such as in the area of immigration policy.

Aging is predominantly a female experience since most older persons are female and women on the average outlive men. Aging policies, however, tend to be based on the male life cycle model and do not account for the gender differences in life trends of employment, health conditions, or family support. Janie S. Steckenrider in "Aging as a Female Phenomenon: The Plight of Older Women" explores the gender bias in existing aging policies and suggests that aging policies need to be more in line with the realities of the population that they serve.

Old-age policy made great advances from the 1930s through the 1970s, for instance; Social Security, Medicare, Medicaid, Supplemental Security Income, and the Older Americans Act, but the politics of retrenchment during the 1980s produced setbacks for many aging policies and led to the politics of "holding on" rather than creating new programs or expanding existing ones. The 1990s brought further shifts in the political climate as the future of old-age policy was threatened by the need to cut spending on costly social programs and by the recurring demands to run a "leaner and meaner" federal government with more state flexibility and individual responsibility. The widespread implications of these federal policy funding dilemmas meant costly and often unbearable consequences for state and local governments, minorities, the elderly, and their families. *New Directions in Old-Age Policies* examines the changed political environment, the implications of these changes on specific aging policy domains, and the challenges of demographic trends and of subgroup populations on aging policy. Our goal is to decipher what this all means for the future of aging policy in the twenty-first century.

References

Liebig, Phoebe S. (1995). Assessing the implications of the 1994 elections for aging policy. *Journal of Aging and Social Policy*, 7(2), 1–11.

Part I

DISTINCT POLICY DOMANS:
A FRESH LOOK AT OLD-AGE POLICIES

Chapter 2

Health Care Policies and Older Americans

ROBERT H. BINSTOCK

In 1995 a Republican-dominated 104th Congress ushered in a new era in the politics of health care policies that affect older Americans. Changes that Congress proposed in Medicare and Medicaid, the major sources of public financing for the health care of older people, involved substantial reductions in projected expenditures and significant structural changes. These proposals were part of a sweeping conservative agenda for limiting the role of government, for redistributing responsibilities of the federal government to state governments, and for bringing the annual federal budget into balance.

Reforms in Medicare, Medicaid, and other health policies relevant to older people have come to the fore on the policy agenda because of two fundamental factors. One is the attempts by federal policymakers to balance the budget, a struggle that is considerably exacerbated by rapidly growing open-ended expenditures in these two entitlement programs. In fiscal 1995, for instance, Medicare and Medicaid outlays combined were estimated to account for 18% of federal spending and were projected to reach 22% by the year 2000 (Congressional Budget Office, 1995a). The other factor is the growth of the older population needing health care, a growth that will accelerate sharply in the early decades of the twenty-first century when the Baby Boom—a cohort of 76 million Americans born between 1946 and 1964—joins the ranks of old age. This demographic phenomenon undergirds dramatic estimates of staggering Medicare and Medicaid expenditures in the future.

During earlier periods in the twentieth century the political context of policies on aging was framed much more by the status of older people and by the efficacy of programs designed to serve them and minor policy reforms had few if any harmful effects on older people. Today the scope of political conflict is much broader and proposed health care policy changes could have considerable adverse consequences for older Americans, especially those who are relatively poor.

This chapter presents an overview of the issues and politics shaping the health care policies that affect older Americans. First, it briefly reviews the costs of health care for older people and how these costs are paid. Second, it considers whether population aging, in itself, is a major factor in the growth of national health care spending. Third, it examines the factors that account for contemporary efforts to curb Medicare expenditures. Fourth, it presents the dilemmas of financing long-term care through Medicaid and other means. It concludes with a brief discussion of the political context that may shape the future of health policies for older Americans.

Financing for Older People's Health Care

Whether or not Congress enacts major changes in Medicare and Medicaid in the late 1990s, health care policies that pay for the care of older people are—and will continue to be—central ingredients in the continuous and major revisions that are taking place in the financing and organization of American health care. Persons aged 65 and older account for roughly one-third of annual U.S. health care costs (U.S. Senate, 1994); in 1994 this amounted to about $300 billion out of $900 billion. Per capita expenditures on older persons are four times greater than on younger persons (Waldo et al., 1989).

Governments fund nearly two-thirds of health care for older Americans. The federal Medicare program, which provides a basic package of health insurance for most Americans who are aged 65 and over (as well as persons who receive federal disability insurance and those with end-stage renal disease), accounts for 45% of the total. Medicaid, jointly funded by the federal and state governments to pay the costs of care for poor people, provides another 12%, principally for long-term care in nursing homes and in other residential environments. Care financed through the Department of Veterans Affairs; the Department of Defense; Indian Health Services; and a variety of other federal, state, and local government programs constitute about 6% of the total. An additional 8% is funded through private insurance, largely from so-called Medigap supplemental policies, and less than 1% comes from philanthropy (U.S. Senate, 1991).

Older persons pay 28% of the costs of their care out-of-pocket. Much of this outlay is for skilled nursing which, along with mental health services, has only minimal Medicare coverage. Nearly two-thirds of prescription drug expenses, not covered at all by Medicare, are paid for out-of-pocket (U.S. Senate, 1994). Persons who can afford Medigap policies have their deductibles and copayments covered reasonably well through insurance. Poor older persons can have their Medicare deductibles and copayments, as well as their Medicare Part B Supplemental Medical Insurance (SMI) premiums, paid by Medicaid through a Qualified Medicare Beneficiary (QMB) program enacted in 1988.

Population Aging and National Health Care Spending

Because the U.S. older population is growing, absolutely and proportionally—from 33 million persons today to an estimated 65 million in the year 2030 (Taeuber, 1992)—health care costs for older persons have frequently been depicted as an unsustainable burden, or as one observer put it, "a great fiscal black hole" that will absorb an unlimited amount of national resources (Callahan, 1987). A report to President Clinton from the Bipartisan Commission on Entitlement and Tax Reform (1994) projected that the proportion of the U.S. Gross Domestic Product (GDP) spent on Medicare and Medicaid would triple between 1993 and 2030, from 3.3% to 11%.

A particular cause for concern is that the population conventionally termed *old* is itself becoming older, and that rates of morbidity and disability are markedly higher at advanced old ages. The number of persons aged 75 and older will grow from 13 million to 30 million between 1990 and 2030, and those aged 85 and older will have increased from 3 million to 8 million (Taueber, 1992). The higher prevalence of morbidity in advanced old ages is reflected in comparative hospitalization rates by age group shown in Table 2.1 where it can be seen, for example, that the rate for persons aged 85 and older is more than triple the rate for persons aged 66 to 69, and over twice the rate for persons aged 70 to 74 (Fortinsky, Binstock, and Rimm, 1994). Similarly, higher prevalence of disability as cohorts reach more advanced old age is manifest in the present rates of nursing home use in different age categories. At present, about 1% of Americans aged 65 to 74 are in nursing homes; this compares with 6.1% of persons aged 75 to 84, and 24% of persons aged 85 and older (U.S. Bureau of the Census, 1993). Disability rates also increase in older old-age categories among elderly persons who are not in nursing homes, from nearly 23% of those aged 65 to 74 to 45% of those aged 85 and older (Cassel, Rudberg, and Olshansky, 1992).

But demography is not destiny with respect to national health care expenditures. U.S. health care spending has increased from less than 6% of GDP in 1965 when Medicare and Medicaid were established (U.S. Senate, 1994), to nearly 15% of GDP today. However, neither increases in the number and proportions of older persons nor the aging of the older population have been major factors in this growth. Demographic factors have been negligible contributors to spiraling health care costs as compared with increases in per capita utilization of services, intensity of services per day or per visit, health-sector specific price inflation, and general inflation (Arnett et al., 1986; Mendelson and Schwartz, 1993; Sonnefeld et al., 1991). If population aging has a major impact on U.S. health care costs, it will not be felt strongly until after 2010 when the Baby Boom begins to join the ranks of persons aged 65 and older; and even this is far from certain.

Table 2.1
Hospitalizations of Medicare Beneficiaries
aged 65 and older, by age group, 1991

Age Group	Percent of Age Group Hospitalized in 1991 (%)
65–69	21.4
70–74	29.6
75–79	37.9
80–84	48.0
85+	63.7
Total 65+	34.1

Source: Fortinsky, Binstock, and Rimm (1994).

In fact, crossnational comparisons of health care expenditures and population aging provide no evidence that substantial and/or rapid population aging causes high levels of national economic burden from expenditures on health care. Health care costs are far from "out of control" or even "high" in many nations that have comparatively large proportions of people aged 65 and older or that have experienced more rapid rates of population aging than the United States. Even when such comparisons are made with respect to more advanced old ages, such as aged 80 and over, there is no apparent relationship with the amount of national wealth spent on health care (Binstock, 1993). The public and private structural features of health care systems (e.g., whether they have relatively fixed or open-ended health care budgets)—and behavioral responses to them by citizens and health care providers—are far more important determinants of a nation's level of health care expenditures than population aging and other demographic trends. The primary reason why the percentage of national wealth spent on health care is far higher in the United States than in any other nation in the world is that much more of U.S. health care is funded on an open-ended basis than in other industrialized nations.

But the structural features of American health care that nourished open-ended funding are undergoing substantial changes as the twentieth century comes to a close. Prominent among these changes are attempts by the federal government to limit spending on the care of older people.

Pressures to Curb Medicare Expenditures

Most of the specific public policy actions and proposals to contain health care costs in recent years have focused on Medicare. There has been no evidence to date that changes in the program have adversely affected the health care or health status of older persons. But efforts to curb federal Medicare expenditures are ongoing and could ultimately have a negative impact on older people.

There are a number of fundamental reasons why Medicare has been a major target in governmental efforts to slow the growth of national health care costs. First, it is the biggest single source of payment for health care in America. Its large aggregate national costs and its rapid inflation are easily determined and highly visible. In 1995 Medicare paid $178 billion for personal health care services and its expenditures are projected to be $288 billion in fiscal year 2000 (Congressional Budget Office, 1995a).

Second, because the federal government pays the bills for Medicare patients, Medicare costs are more directly responsive to government action than those paid by private insurance and out-of-pocket. The most far-reaching cost-containment measures undertaken to date have been changes in reimbursement procedures under Medicare, such as prospective payment on the basis of diagnosis-related groups to control expenditures on hospitals (Coulam and Gaumer, 1991), the introduction of a "resource based relative-value scale" for reimbursing physicians, and the introduction of Medicare HMOs (health maintenance organizations) (Brown et al., 1993).

Third, changes in Medicare approaches to paying for care are a plausible strategy for implementing the more general goal of cost-containment. This nationwide governmental program affects the financial incentives of most American hospitals, nursing homes, physicians, and other health care providers and suppliers. Consequently, changes in Medicare have impacts on the overall health care arena that extend beyond the provision of services to Medicare patients.

Fourth, the issue of how to pay for Medicare is rather immediate. Recent annual reports of the Trustees of the Social Security Trust Funds have consistently estimated that in the latter half of the 1990s the funds will run a deficit. Annual expenditures for Medicare's Part A Hospital Insurance (HI) already exceed substantially the revenues from the payroll tax that finances it, and HI trust fund reserves are being drawn upon to bridge the gap. A mid-1996 report of the Trustees of the Social Security Trust Fund estimated that the fund's reserves will be exhausted early in 2001 (Rosenbaum, 1996). Moreover, the financing of Medicare's Part B nonhospital Supplemental Medical Insurance (SMI) has moved from being principally financed by premiums from Medicare enrollees, as in the early years of the program, to being three-quarters financed from general revenues, today. As SMI expenditures increase (presently at a rate that is 50% faster than spending on Part A), so does the amount of general revenues needed to support them. The Omnibus Budget Reconciliation Act (OBRA) of 1993 partially responded to these immediate issues by enacting Medicare spending reductions and revenue increases totaling an estimated $85 billion over the five-year period 1994–98 (Congressional Budget Office, 1993). But these measures have not been sufficient to eliminate the near-term financing problem in Part A or the growing pressure on general revenues to meet rapidly expanding Part B expenses.

Finally, as implied by spending projections, Medicare could contribute substantially to increases in the federal deficit in the years to come unless significant changes are made in the program (Congressional Budget Office, 1995b). Consequently, as national policymakers become increasingly serious about balancing the budget, their attention is inevitably drawn to limiting the growth of financing for Medicare.

In the fall of 1995 the Republican-dominated 104th Congress submitted to President Clinton a budget bill for fiscal year 1996 that included a $270-billion reduction in projected Medicare spending by 2002. The Democratic president vetoed the bill, citing the size of the Medicare reduction and the structural changes proposed for the program as among his reasons for doing so.

By mid-1996 Congress had yet to submit a new budget bill. It was unclear whether Medicare spending reductions and structural reforms would be enacted at all during the 104th Congress. Nonetheless, there was a consensus among the political parties that major savings in Medicare should be enacted, regardless of the specific amount. The president was proposing to slow the growth of Part A expenditures by $72 billion by the year 2002; the Republican leadership was setting a target of $123 billion over the same period (Wines, 1996). With new projections by the Congressional Budget Office and an increased emphasis on deficit reduction, in 1997 the president and the Republicans reached an agreement to slow the growth in Medicare Part A spending by $115 billion over five years, essentially "splitting the difference" between the most recent offers from both sides. The strategies envisioned for achieving reductions are likely to shape the agenda for Medicare reform for the rest of the decade.

The general approach that appears to be favored is a transition from Medicare's traditional open-ended fee-for-service approach to paying for health care to a situation in which most of Medicare operates with fixed budgets that cap program costs. The various strategies envisioned for carrying out this approach pose some possible adverse consequences for segments of the older population.

One strategy is to encourage both the proliferation of, and enrollment in, Medicare managed care plans that receive a flat per capita fee for providing health care for each beneficiary enrolled in the plan. The financial incentives of managed care organizations, however, foster undertreatment of patients (see Kane and Kane, 1994). Nothing in the experience of over a decade of Medicare HMO experiments launched by the federal Health Care Financing

Administration is reassuring on this score, because enrollees in these programs have tended to be relatively healthy older persons (see Brown et al., 1993), and even they seem to have been underserved in certain respects (Wiener and Skaggs, 1995).

A second strategy is to establish individual tax-exempt Medical Savings Accounts (MSAs) through which each Medicare participant would receive an annual flat sum from Medicare, be required to use part of it to purchase a high-deductible catastrophic health insurance policy, and use the balance (if he or she chooses) to purchase health care. Unused balances in such accounts would be retained by Medicare participants, spent or invested by them, and could even be passed on through inheritance. Most policy analysts expect that relatively healthy and wealthy older people would opt for MSAs. But it is also a distinct possibility that poorer older people would select the MSA option, too. The sum paid into MSAs by Medicare may be perceived as a substantial cash windfall by older people who are either below the poverty line or only a few thousand dollars above it. Those poorer people who elect the MSA may well forego needed medical care in order to preserve the windfall, even though poorer old people tend to be relatively unhealthy (Robert and House, 1994).

A third strategy is to set a projected annual spending cap for aggregate reimbursements for the traditional fee-for-service portion of Medicare. If spending exceeds the cap, a "fail-safe" mechanism would enforce the target by reducing reimbursement rates to health care providers in order to make up for the aggregate excess spending. This, in turn, would likely have an impact on the quality of care received by Medicare patients.

The Dilemmas of Financing Long-Term Care

Although the contemporary policy agenda with respect to Medicare is essentially one of cutting government costs, the issues of resource allocation for long-term care are more complex. Out-of-pocket payments are large and unaffordable for many. Private insurance is expensive and limited in coverage. Medicaid plays a key role in financing long-term care for poor people and for those who become poor through paying for their care out-of-pocket; but the program is an increasing cost for federal and state governments. A few years ago it seemed that the federal government might expand public funding for long-term care by creating a new insurance program. Now, however, policymakers are attempting to cut back on Medicaid spending and to find new models for delivering Medicaid-financed care within the context of fixed budgets.

Overall Costs

Expenditures for long-term care of older people are substantial and very likely to increase in the decades immediately ahead. The total bill in 1993 was $75.5 billion; 72% was spent on nursing home care and 28% on home and community-based care (Wiener, Illston, and Hanley, 1994). Out-of-pocket payments by individuals and their families account for 44% of the total. Only 1% is paid for with private insurance benefits. The remaining 55% is financed by federal, state, and local governments.

The demand for long-term care of older people will increase considerably in the twenty-first century. As noted earlier, the number of people aged 65 and older will have more than doubled between 1990 and 2030 (Taeuber, 1992). Experts disagree as to whether rates of disability in old age will increase or decline in the future. But even those who report a decline in the prevalence of disability at older ages in recent years emphasize that there will be large absolute increases in the number of older Americans needing long-term care in the decades ahead (see, e.g., Manton, Corder, and Stallard, 1993). Accordingly, the Congressional Budget Office (1991), using 1990 as a baseline year, projects that total national costs of long-term care will almost double by 2010 and more than triple by 2030.

The Role of Individuals and Their Families

Many persons needing formal, paid long-term care services have no way to pay for them. In one study, for example, about 75% of unpaid, informal caregivers of dementia patients said that they did not use paid services because they could not afford them (Eckert and Smyth, 1988). Although dozens of governmental programs provide funding for long-term care services (U.S. General Accounting Office, 1995), many persons needing long-term care are ineligible for these programs.

Although nearly half of the national bill for long-term care is paid for out-of-pocket, such payments are a significant financial burden for many individuals and their families. The annual cost of a year's care in a nursing home averages $37,000 (Wiener and

Illston, 1996) and ranges higher than $100,000. While the use of a limited number of services in a home or other community-based setting is less expensive, noninstitutional care for patients who would otherwise be appropriately placed in a nursing home is not cheaper and often is more expensive (Weissert, 1990).

A number of research efforts have documented that about 80% of the long-term care provided to older persons outside of nursing homes is presently provided on an in-kind basis by family members—spouses, siblings, adult children, and broader kin networks (see chapter by Parrott in this volume). About 74% of dependent community-based older persons receive all their care from family members or from other unpaid sources: about 21% receive both formal and informal services; and only about 5% use just formal services (Liu, Manton, and Liu, 1985). The vast majority of family caregivers are women (see Brody, 1990; Stone, Cafferata, and Sangl, 1987). The family also plays an important role in obtaining and managing services from paid service providers.

The capacities and willingness of family members to care for disabled older persons may decline, however, when the Baby Boom cohort reaches old age because of a broad social trend. The family, as a fundamental unit of social organization, has been undergoing profound transformations that will become more fully manifest over the next few decades as Baby Boomers reach old age. The striking growth of single-parent households, the growing participation of women in the labor force, and the high incidence of divorce and remarriage (differentially higher for men), all entail complicated changes in the structure of household and kinship roles and relationships. There will be an increasing number of "blended families," reflecting multiple lines of descent through multiple marriages and the birth of children outside of wedlock through other partners. This growth in the incidence of step- and half-relatives will make for a dramatic new turn in family structure in the coming decades. Already, such blended families constitute about half of all households with children (National Academy on Aging, 1994).

One possible implication of these changes is that kinship networks in the near future will become more complex, attenuated, and diffuse (Bengtson, Rosenthal, and Burton, 1990), perhaps with a weakened sense of filial obligation. If changes in the intensity of kinship relations significantly erode the capacity and sense of obligation to care for older family members when the Baby Boom cohort is in the ranks of old age and disability, demands for governmental support to pay long-term care may increase accordingly (see chapter by Parrott in this volume).

The Role of Private Insurance

Although Medicare pays for short-term, subacute nursing care, it does not reimburse patients for long-term care, either in nursing homes or at home. Private long-term care insurance, a relatively new product, is very expensive for the majority of older persons and its benefits are limited in scope and duration. The best quality policies—providing substantial benefits over a reasonable period of time—charged premiums in 1991 that averaged $2,525 for persons aged 65 and $7,675 for those aged 79 (Wiener and Illston, 1996). About 4% to 5% of older persons have any private long-term care insurance and only about 1% of nursing home costs are paid by private insurance (Wiener, Illston, and Hanley, 1994). A number of analyses have suggested that even when the product becomes more refined, no more than 20% of older Americans will be able to afford it (Crown, Capitman, and Leutz, 1992; Friedland, 1990; Rivlin and Wiener, 1988; Wiener, Illston, and Hanley, 1994). Although some studies suggest a potential for a higher percentage of customers, they assume relatively limited packages of benefit coverage (e.g., Cohen et al., 1987).

A variation on the private insurance policy approach to financing long-term care is continuing care retirement communities (CCRCs) which promise comprehensive health care services—including long-term care—to all members (Chellis and Grayson, 1990). CCRC customers tend to be middle- and upper-income persons who are relatively healthy when they become residents and who pay a substantial entrance charge and monthly fee in return for a promise of "care for life." It has been estimated that about 10% of older people could afford to join such communities (Cohen, 1988). Most of the 1,000 CCRCs in the United States, however, do not provide complete benefit coverage in their contracts, and those that do have faced financial difficulties (Williams and Temkin-Greener, 1996). Because most older people prefer to remain in their own homes rather than join age-segregated communities, an alternative product termed *life care at home* (LCAH) was developed in the late 1980s and was marketed to middle-income customers with lower entry and monthly fees than those of CCRCs (Tell, Cohen, and Wallack, 1987). There are, however, only about 500 LCAH policies in effect (Williams and Temkin-Greener, 1996).

A relatively new approach for providing long-term care in residential settings is the "assisted living" facility. It has been created for moderately disabled persons—including those with dementia—who are not ready for a nursing home, and provides them with limited forms of personal care, supervision of medications and other daily routines, and congregate meal and housekeeping services (Kane and Wilson, 1993; Regnier, Hamilton, and Yatabe, 1995). Assisted living has yet to be tried with a private insurance approach. The monthly rent in a first-class nonprofit facility averages about $2,400 for a one-bedroom apartment; the rent is higher in for-profit facilities.

The Role of Medicaid

For those who cannot pay for long-term care out-of-pocket or through various insurance arrangements, and who are not eligible for care through programs of the Department of Veterans Affairs, the available sources of payment are Medicaid and other means-tested government programs funded by the Older Americans Act, Social Service Block Grants (Title XX of the Social Security Act), and state and local governments. The bulk of such financing is through Medicaid that paid an estimated 52% of total national nursing home expenditures in 1993, accounting for one-quarter of all Medicaid spending (Burner, Waldo, and McKusick, 1992).

Medicaid, the federal-state program for the poor, finances the care—at least in part—of about three-fifths of nursing home patients (Wiener and Illston, 1996) and 28% of home and community-based services (American Association of Retired Persons, 1994). The program does not pay for the full range of home care services that are needed for most clients who are functionally dependent. Most state Medicaid programs provide reimbursement only for the most "medicalized" services that are necessary to maintain a long-term care patient in a home environment; rarely reimbursed are essential supports such as chore services, assistance with food shopping and meal preparation, transportation, companionship, periodic monitoring, and respite programs for family and other unpaid caregivers.

Medicaid does include a special waiver program that allows states to offer a wider range of nonmedical home care services, if limited to those patients whose services will be no more costly than Medicaid-financed nursing home care. But the volume of services in these waiver programs—which in some states combine Medicaid with funds from the Older Americans Act, the Social Services Block Grant program, and other state and local government sources—is small in relation to the overall demand (Miller, 1992).

Although many patients are poor enough to qualify for Medicaid when they enter a nursing home, a substantial number become poor after they are institutionalized (Adams, Meiners, and Burwell, 1993). Persons in this latter group deplete their assets in order to meet their bills and eventually "spend down" and become poor enough to qualify for Medicaid.

Still others become eligible for Medicaid by sheltering their assets—illegally or legally with the assistance of attorneys who specialize in so-called Medicaid Estate Planning. Because sheltered assets are not counted in Medicaid eligibility determinations, such persons are able to take advantage of a program for the poor, without being poor. Asset sheltering has become a source of considerable concern to the federal and state governments as Medicaid expenditures on nursing homes are increasing rapidly—projected to triple from 1990 to 2000 (Burner, Waldo, and McKusick, 1992).

An analysis in Virginia estimated that the aggregate of assets sheltered through the use of legal loopholes in 1991 was equal to more than 10% of what the state spent on nursing home care through Medicaid in that year (Burwell, 1993). A study drawing on interviews with state government staff for Medicaid eligibility determination in four states—California, Florida, Massachusetts, and New York—found a strong relationship between a high level of financial wealth in a geographic area and a high level of Medicaid estate planning activity. Most of these workers estimated that the range of asset sheltering among single applicants for Medicaid was between 5% and 10%, and for married applicants, between 20% and 25% (Burwell and Crown, 1995).

Efforts to Expand and Contract Public Funding

From the mid-1980s until the mid-1990s a number of national policymakers were sympathetic to these various dilemmas—the inability of individuals and their families to pay for services, the limitations of private insurance, and the anxieties of spending down. Since then, however, the main concern in Washington, as well as in the states, has been to limit Medicaid expenditures. In this new context, the most likely prospect is that public resources for long-term care will be even less available, in relation to the need, than they have been to date.

In the early 1990s advocates for the elderly, as well as younger disabled persons, were optimistic that the federal government would establish a new program for public long-term care insurance that would not be means-tested as is Medicaid. A number of bills introduced from 1989 to 1994 included some version of such a program, including President Clinton's failed proposal for health care reform (see Binstock, 1994). None of these proposals became law. The major reason was that any substantial version of such a program would cost tens of billions of dollars each year just at the outset, and far more as the Baby Boom reaches old age.

By 1995, however, legislative focus had shifted from creating a new program to curbing the costs of public expenditures for long-term care. Medicaid's expenditures on long-term care had been growing at an annualized rate of 13.2% since 1989 (U.S. General Accounting Office, 1995).

As part of its overall effort to achieve a balanced budget by 2002, Congress initially proposed in the summer of 1995 to cap the rate of growth in Medicaid expenditures in order to achieve savings of $182 billion, to eliminate federal requirements for determining individual eligibility for Medicaid (as an entitlement), and to turn over control of the program to state governments through capped block grants. Late in the year Clinton vetoed a budget bill that contained such changes. But the reductions and structural changes proposed by Congress remained on the policy agenda, supported by the National Governors Conference.

According to one analysis (Kassner, 1995), the 1995 congressional proposals for limiting Medicaid's growth would have trimmed long-term care funding by as much as 11.4% by 2000 and meant that 1.74 million Medicaid beneficiaries would have lost or been unable to secure coverage. In addition, this analysis assumed that states would make their initial reductions in home and community-based care services (because nursing home residents have nowhere else to go), and concluded that such services would be substantially reduced from their current levels. Five states were projected to completely eliminate home and community-based services by the end of the century and another nineteen to cut services by more than half. Whether or not these specific predictions come true, if provisions to cap and block-grant Medicaid do become law, they will almost certainly engender conflict within states regarding the distribution of limited resources for the care of older and younger poor constituencies.

Experimental Programs

Meanwhile, a number of experiments in new ways to finance and deliver long-term care have been underway. These experiments—sponsored by private foundations and state governments, as well as by the federal government—have been attempting to demonstrate that appropriate long-term care can be delivered in fashions that limit out-of-pocket and governmental expenditures, and effectively integrate acute and long-term health care.

PRIVATE INSURANCE/MEDICAID PARTNERSHIPS. The Robert Wood Johnson Foundation has undertaken experimental programs in four states intended to enable middle- and upper-income older persons to protect their assets from being spent down and yet have Medicaid pay for their long-term care (Meiners, 1996). At the same time these programs are designed to reduce the period that Medicaid needs to finance the care of individuals whose services are reduced by the program.

Through this Partnership for Long-Term Care Program, state governments agree to exempt individuals who apply for Medicaid eligibility from having to spend down assets in order to qualify for the program, if they have previously had some long-term care paid for by a state-certified private insurance policy. In California, Connecticut, and Indiana, the Medicaid agencies will allow a dollar of asset protection for each dollar that has been paid by insurance. In New York, after three years of private insurance coverage for nursing home services or six months of home health care, protection is granted for all assets although the individual's income must be devoted to the cost of care along with Medicaid. This experiment is in its early stages and cannot yet be evaluated.

FINANCING THROUGH INTEGRATION WITH ACUTE CARE. Experimental models have also been developed for financing long-term care services by integrating them with acute care. These models are being refined through field demonstrations. Each involves mechanisms of managed care. But their differences illustrate some of the issues and challenges generated by various sources of funding and by different types of older patient populations.

A model initially tested at several sites in the 1980s is the Social/Health Maintenance Organization (S/HMO), financed by the federal government. The S/HMO offers customers a limited package of home and community-based long-term care benefits on a capitated basis as a supplement to Medicare HMO benefits, and attempts to enroll primarily healthy older customers (Leutz et al., 1985). Results from these early experiments were equivocal with respect to the viability of financing arrangements and target populations (Newcomer, Harrington, and Friedlob, 1990). Consequently,

Congress has called for a second round of S/HMO demonstrations to test refinements such as heavy involvement of geriatricians and geriatric nurse practitioners; standard protocols for obtaining adequate medical and social histories, and for diagnosing and managing conditions frequently found in older patients; increased attention to the effects of prescription drugs on patients; and outpatient alternatives to hospitalization and nursing home placement.

While the S/HMO attempts to enroll healthy older persons to demonstrate what is feasible financially with such a population, the On Lok model, developed at a San Francisco neighborhood center in the 1970s and early 1980s, is targeted to community-based older persons who are already sufficiently dependent in daily functioning to be appropriately placed in a nursing home. In this capitated model most patients are eligible for both Medicare and Medicaid. Services are organized around an adult day care program that not only serves as a social program and as a respite for caregivers, but also functions much like a geriatric outpatient clinic with substantial medical observation and supervision (Zawadski and Eng, 1988).

The On Lok model, now being replicated at ten demonstration sites as a Program for All-Inclusive Care for the Elderly (PACE), appears to have integrated acute and long-term care fairly well under its managed care approach. Whether it can be extended beyond the very frail population it has served to date—patients who are already functionally dependent, and dually eligible for Medicare and Medicaid—remains to be seen. (To some extent, this is what is being explored in the second round of the S/HMO demonstrations.) Early evaluations of the PACE demonstrations indicate that they are experiencing problems of financial viability, high staff turnover among physicians and adult day health center directors, and in getting the right patient mix in terms of both acuity and dementia (Kane, Illston, and Miller, 1992).

Still another model for attempting to integrate the financing and delivery of acute and long-term care for older persons is the Minnesota Long-Term Care Options Project (LTCOP). It incorporates elements of both the S/HMO and On Lok models. In contrast to the S/HMO, however, the LTCOP will target Medicaid eligible enrollees and accordingly offer a benefit package that includes nursing home care as well as home and community-based care. It will also include a less functionally dependent population than the On Lok model. Hence, it provides an opportunity to test broader approaches to integrating acute and long-term care than have been tried to date.

To the extent that any of these demonstration models seem to be effective in integrating care as they are tested in the years immediately ahead, their broader import in the American health care delivery system for older adults will still depend upon further action by the federal government and in the private sector. The government would need to allow the pooling of Medicare and Medicaid funds more generally for this purpose (the various demonstration models operate under special waivers from the Health Care Financing Administration that administers these two programs). And to make such care integration available for those older persons not covered by Medicaid for long-term care expenses, private insurance companies will need to be satisfied that such managed care arrangements are financially viable.

Table 2.2 summarizes the long-term care experimental programs.

Conclusion

A new era in the politics of aging is emerging. Proposals for major changes in health policies affecting older Americans have been generated by conservative political principles and by efforts to balance the federal budget, without much attention to the implications for older people, themselves. These changes will stay on the policy agenda for some time to come because of enormous projected future costs of the Medicare and Medicaid programs. If the kinds of reforms that were contemplated in 1995 for substantially re-

Table 2.2
Long-Term Care Experimental Programs

Private Insurance/Medicaid Partnerships	—Partnership for Long-Term Care, Robert Wood Johnson Foundation
Integration with Acute Care	—S/HMO (Social Health Maintenance Organization) —On Lok Model/PACE (Program for All-Inclusive Care for the Elderly) —LTCOP (Minnesota Long-Term Care Options Projects)

structuring and reducing projected expenditures in these two programs are enacted, they are likely to have unfortunate consequences for older persons, particularly those among them who are relatively poor.

Although old-age-based interest groups—the so-called gray lobby (Pratt, 1976)—are reputed to be politically powerful, they are unlikely to have much impact in their efforts to fend off major changes in Medicare and Medicaid. The key actions among those taken by the old-age groups will be those of the American Association for Retired Persons (AARP). In addition to the implicit political bluff of having thirty-three million members of voting age AARP has substantial financial resources to undergird its political activities, including an annual income that approaches $500 million (see chapter by Day in this volume). In recent years, however, including 1995 when Congress attempted to reform Medicare and Medicaid, AARP has chosen moderate political strategies in attempts to counter what it regards as undesirable policy changes in programs on aging (Binstock, 1995).

AARP is likely to continue to choose moderate political strategies in the years immediately ahead. The major reason is that it will be guided by the fundamental imperative of organizational survival. From the perspective of the classic literature on political organizations (Clark and Wilson, 1961; Wilson, 1973) AARP is an organization that maintains itself primarily through the material and associational incentives that it provides to its members, rather than political incentives. Seen in this light, the political activities of AARP can be interpreted as membership marketing strategies. In short, the incentive system of the organization tends to dictate that it should clearly establish a record that it is fighting to defend against major changes in old-age programs. But this fight, win or lose, should not include controversial positions and tactics that threaten to jeopardize the stability of the organization's membership and financial resources.

Consequently, the old-age lobby is unlikely to have much impact on proposed reforms in Medicare, Medicaid, and other health programs for older people. The future of American health policy is much more likely to be shaped by vested interests in the health care industry, broader business interests, and whether a congressional majority and a president can eventually agree on details of program revisions. One thing is certain: Medicare and Medicaid will be changed substantially over the next twenty years as the Baby Boom begins to join the ranks of old age.

References

Adams, E. K., Meiners, M. R., and Burwell, B. O. (1993). Asset spend-down in nursing homes: Methods and insights. *Medical Care*, 31, 1–23.

American Association of Retired Persons (AARP), Public Policy Institute. (1994). *The Costs of Long-term Care*. Washington, DC: AARP.

Arnett, R. H., III, McKusick, D. R., Sonnefeld, S. T., and Cowell, C. S. (1986). Projections of health care spending to 1990. *Health Care Financing Review*, 7 (3), 1–36.

Bengtson, V. L., Rosenthal, C., and Burton, L. (1990). Families and aging: Diversity and heterogeneity. In R. H. Binstock and L. K. George (Eds.), *Handbook of Aging and the Social Sciences*. 3rd ed., pp. 263–87. San Diego, CA: Academic.

Binstock, R. H. (1993). Health care costs around the world: Is aging a fiscal "black hole"? *Generations*, 17 (4), 37–42.

———. (1994). Older Americans and health care reform in the 1990s. In P. V. Rosenau (Ed.), *Health Care Reform in the Nineties*, pp. 213–35. Thousand Oaks, CA: Sage Publications.

———. (1995). A new era in the politics of aging: How will the old-age interest groups respond? *Generations*, 19 (3), 68–74.

Bipartisan Commission on Entitlement and Tax Reform. (1994). *Interim Report to the President*. Washington, DC: U.S. Government Printing Office.

Brody, E. M. (1990). *Women in the Middle: Their Parent-Care Years*. New York: Springer Publishing.

Brown, R. S., Bergeron, J. W., Clement, D. G., Hill, J. W., and Retchin, S. M. (1993). *Does Managed Care Work for Medicare? An Evaluation of the Medicare Risk Program for HMOs*. Princeton, NJ: Mathematica.

Burner, S. T., Waldo, D. R., and McKusick, D. R. (1992). National health expenditures projections through 2030. *Health Care Financing Review*, 14 (1), 1–29.

Burwell, B. (1993). *State Responses to Medicaid Estate Planning*. Cambridge, MA: SysteMetrics.

Burwell, B., and Crown, W. H. (1995). Medicaid estate planning in the aftermath of OBRA '93. Cambridge, MA: MEDSTAT Group.

Callahan, D. (1987). *Setting Limits: Medical Goals in an Aging Society*. New York: Simon & Schuster.

Cassel, C. K., Rudberg, M. A., and Olshansky, S. J. (1992). The price of success: Health care in an aging society. *Health Affairs*, 11 (2), 87–99.

Chellis, R. D., and Grayson, P. J. (1990). *Life Care: A Long-term Solution?* Lexington, MA: Lexington Books.

Clark, P. B., and Wilson, J. Q. (1961). Incentive systems: A theory of organizations. *Administrative Science Quarterly*, 6, 219–66.

Cohen, M. A. (1988). Life care: New options for financing and delivering long-term care. *Health Care Financing Review, Annual Supplement*, 139–43.

Cohen, M. A., Tell, E., Greenberg, J., and Wallack, S. S. (1987). The financial capacity of the elderly to insure for long-term care. *Gerontologist*, 27, 494–502.

Congressional Budget Office, Congress of the United States. (1991). *Policy Choices for Long-term Care*. Washington, DC: U.S. Government Printing Office.

———. (1993). *The Economic and Budget Outlook: An Update*. Washington, DC: U.S. Government Printing Office.

———. (1995a). *The Economic and Budget Outlook: An Update*. Washington, DC: U.S. Government Printing Office.

———. (1995b). *The Economic and Budget Outlook: Fiscal Years 1996–2000*. Washington, DC: U.S. Government Printing Office.

Coulam, R. F., and Gaumer, G. L. (1991). Medicare's prospective payment system: A critical appraisal. *Health Care Financing Review, Annual Supplement*, 45–77.

Crown, W. H, Capitman, J., and Leutz, W. N. (1992). Economic rationality, the affordability of private long-term care insurance, and the role for public policy. *Gerontologist*, 32, 478–85.

Eckert, S. K., and Smyth, K. (1988). *A Case Study of Methods of Locating and Arranging Health and Long-term Care for Persons with Dementia*. Washington, DC: Office of Technology Assessment, Congress of the United States.

Fortinsky, R. H., Binstock, R. H., and Rimm, A. A. (1994). Some age-based rationing scenarios: How much money would be saved? Paper presented at the 122nd Annual Meeting of the American Public Health Association, Washington, DC, 3 November.

Friedland, R. (1990). *Facing the Costs of Long-term Care: An EBRI-ERF Policy Study*. Washington, DC: Employee Benefits Research Institute.

Kane, R. L., and Kane, R. A. (1994). Effects of the Clinton health reform on older persons and their families: A health care systems perspective. *Gerontologist*, 34, 598–605.

Kane, R. A., and Wilson, K. B. (1993). *Assisted Living in the United States: A New Paradigm for Residential Care for Older People?* Washington, DC: AARP.

Kane, R. L., Illston, L. H., and Miller, N. A. (1992). Qualitative analysis of the Program of All-inclusive Care for the Elderly (PACE). *Gerontologist*, 32, 771–80.

Kassner, E. (1995). *Long-term Care: Measuring the Impact of a Medicaid Cap.* Washington, DC: Public Policy Institute, AARP.

Leutz, W., Greenberg, J. N., Abrahams, R., Prottas, J., Diamond L. M., and Gruenberg, L. (1985). *Changing Health Care for an Aging Society: Planning for the Social/Health Maintenance Organization.* Lexington, MA: Lexington Books.

Liu, K., Manton, K. M., and Liu, B. M. (1985). Home care expenses for the disabled elderly. *Health Care Financing Review*, 7 (2), 51–58.

Manton, K. G., Corder, L. S., and Stallard, E. (1993). Estimates of change in chronic disability and institutional incidence and prevalence rates in the U.S. elderly population from the 1982, 1984, and 1989 National Long-Term Care Survey. *Journal of Gerontology: Social Sciences*, 48, S153–S166.

Meiners, M. R. (1996). The financing and organization of long-term care. In R. H. Binstock, L. E. Cluff, and O. von Mering (Eds.), *The Future of Long-term Care: Social and Policy Issues*, pp. 191–214. Baltimore, MD: Johns Hopkins University Press.

Mendelson, D. N., and Schwartz, W. B. (1993). The effects of aging and population growth on health care costs. *Health Affairs*, 12 (1), 119–25.

Miller, N. A. (1992). Medicaid 2176 home and community-based care waivers: The first ten years. *Health Affairs*, 11 (4), 162–71.

National Academy on Aging. (1994). *Old Age in the 21st Century.* Washington, DC: Syracuse University Press.

Newcomer, R. J., Harrington, C., and Friedlob, A. (1990). Social health maintenance organizations: Assessing their initial experience. *Health Services Research*, 25, 425–54.

Pratt, H. J. (1976). *The Gray Lobby.* Chicago: University of Chicago Press.

Regnier, V., Hamilton, J., and Yatabe, S. (1995). *Assisted Living for the Aged and Frail: Innovations in Design, Management, and Financing.* New York: Columbia University Press.

Rivlin, A. M., and Wiener, J. M. (1988). *Caring for the Disabled Elderly: Who Will Pay?* Washington, DC: Brookings Institution.

Robert, S. A., and House, J. S. (1994). Socioeconomic status and health over the life course. In R. A. Abeles, H. C. Gift, and M. G. Ory (Eds.), *Aging and the Quality of Life,* pp. 253–74. New York: Springer Publishing.

Rosenbaum, David E. (1996). Gloomy forecast touches off feud on Medicare fund. *New York Times,* 6 June, p. 1.

Sonnenfeld, S. T., Waldo, D. R., Lemieux, J., and McKusick, D. R. (1991). Projections of national health expenditures through the year 2000. *Health Care Financing Review,* 13 (1), 1–27.

Stone, R., Cafferata, G. L., and Sangl, J. (1987). Caregivers of the frail elderly: A national profile. *Gerontologist,* 27, 616–26.

Taeuber, C. M. (1992). *Sixty-five Plus in America.* U.S. Department of Commerce, Bureau of the Census, Current Populations Reports, Special Studies, P23–178. Washington, DC: U.S. Government Printing Office.

Tell, E. J., Cohen, M. A., and Wallack, S. S. (1987). New directions in lifecare: An industry in transition. *Milbank Quarterly,* 65, 551–74.

U.S. Bureau of the Census. (1993). *Nursing Home Population: 1990.* CPH-L-137. Washington, DC: U.S. Government Printing Office.

U.S. General Accounting Office. (1995). *Long-term Care: Current Issues and Future Directions.* Washington, DC: U.S. Government Printing Office.

U.S. Senate, Special Committee on Aging. (1991). *Aging America: Trends and Projections.* Washington, DC: U.S. Government Printing Office.

———. (1994). *Developments in Aging: 1993,* Vol. 1. Washington, DC: U.S. Government Printing Office.

Waldo, D. R., Sonnefeld, S. T., McKusick, D. R., and Arnett, R. H. (1989). Health expenditures by age group, 1977 and 1987. *Health Care Financing Review,* 10 (4), 111–20.

Weissert, W. G. (1990). Strategies for reducing home care expenditures. *Generations,* 14 (2), 42–44.

M., and Illston, L. H. (1996). Health care financing and organi-
for the elderly. In R. H. Binstock and L. K. George (Eds.),
of *Aging and the Social Sciences, Fourth Edition,* pp.
n Diego, CA: Academic.

Chapter 3

Economic Security: Strengthening Social Security

YUNG-PING CHEN

The retirement income system in the United States has frequently been symbolized as a three-legged stool: Social Security providing a floor of income protection with supplements from private pensions and individual savings. According to the latest available statistics (1994), of those aged 65 and over, 91% received Social Security and 42% of their income came from it; 30% received private pension and 10% of their income came from it; 67% received asset income and 18% of their income came from it; and 21% had employment and 18% of their income was from earnings (Grad, 1996).

It is evident that Social Security is the most important source of income for older persons. After reviewing the relative roles of various income sources, this chapter discusses the ideas for reforming Social Security.

Relative Roles and Current Status of Income Sources

Social Security

A social insurance program, Social Security was enacted in 1935 to provide old-age benefits. It was expanded to include survivors benefits in 1939 and disability benefits in 1956. These three components, old-age, survivors, and disability insurance (OASDI) constitute what is meant by Social Security. Over the last thirty years, it has continued to gain in importance as an income source

37

for older persons. In 1962, 69% of the aged received income from Social Security, compared to 91% in 1994. The contribution of Social Security to the total income of the older population has also grown, accounting for 31% in 1962 to 42% in 1994.

Social Security maintains two trust funds, one for the old-age and survivors insurance (OASI) and the other for the disability insurance (DI). Generally, OASDI trust funds are discussed together. Although the trust funds currently have a reserve of approximately $500 billion and are projected to grow for a number of years, OASDI Board of Trustees (1996) indicates that the program is actuarially sound in the short range (10 years) but not in the long range (75 years). Under the intermediate (best guess) assumptions, the long-range actuarial deficit for the period 1996 through 2070 is estimated at 2.19% of taxable payroll. The board also estimates that the OASDI trust funds will be exhausted in the year 2029.

Even with trust fund exhaustion, Social Security will not cease to exist because there still will be tax revenue based on the 12.4% payroll tax rate (evenly divided by employees and employers alike). However, the revenue will be insufficient to pay all the benefits on a timely basis as promised under present law. For example, based on intermediate assumptions, the tax revenue in 2029 will only amount to 77% of what will be required to pay benefits in full to everyone for that year. How to deal with the deficit problem is a pressing issue discussed in the following section.

Private Pensions

Private pensions as an income source have grown significantly since 1950 when pension plans first became accepted as a proper issue for collective bargaining as a result of the Supreme Court decision in the 1949 *Inland Steel* case. Private pensions have also gained in relative importance in the last three decades. In 1962 only 9% of older people had private pension income, while 30% did in 1994. The relative importance of this income source has likewise increased, accounting for 5% of their total income in 1962 and 10% in 1994 (Grad, 1996).

Although there is a trend in recent years toward greater pension receipt rates, especially for women and minorities, a confluence of developments in the economy and the labor market does not bode well for the future of private pensions as a source of retirement income for many (Chen, 1995b; see chapter by Steckenrider in this volume). First, the decrease in the proportion of workers in manufacturing and the rising percentage of workers in low-paying service jobs imply less pension participation, because pensions are less prevalent in service fields than in industry. Second, the growing importance of (voluntary) part-time employment and the movement toward "contracting out" or "outsourcing" of work suggest that a lower percentage of the work force will be eligible for the retirement benefits earned by full-time employees.

Third, the movement from defined-benefit to defined-contribution pension plans will result in less predictable retirement income. With defined-contribution plans, investment risk shifts to the employee, making future benefit levels more uncertain. And fourth, the downsizing of corporate America in recent years has compressed the ranks of middle management, just as women and minorities were making their way to that tier of business. All of this points to a future in which the role of private pensions in providing retirement income may be even less dependable than it is at present.

Asset Income

In the past three decades, income from assets has increased its role in older persons' total income. While 54% of the elderly population received income from assets in 1962, 67% of them did in 1994. This income source also became a larger share of the total income of older persons, increasing from 16% in 1962 to 18% in 1994. For the highest income group, asset income is the most important source (Grad, 1996). The median amounts of asset income were quite low. One major reason is the typically small or modest value of the elderly's liquid or financial assets (Radner, 1988).

Another problem is the nonliquid nature of home equity. About 75% of the elderly are homeowners, and about 80% of them own their homes without mortgage debt. Homeownership represents considerable wealth; some 70% of the elderly's total assets is their home equity. Home equity is the current market value of the house minus the existing mortgage, if any. Home equity yields little or no spendable cash, and because of it, may be considered a "frozen" asset.

However, home equity could possibly be "liquified" through various methods to convert it into currently spendable cash, methods involving a loan or a sale that allows occupancy. Home Equity Liquifying Plans (HELP) may appeal to those who prefer to generate more income without relinquishing occupancy in the house. HELP would complement long-term health care at home when homecare is feasible and desired (Chen, 1995a; see chapter by Liebig in this volume).

Although converting home equity to currently spendable cash on a voluntary basis could enhance the income position of many elderly homeowners, this financial option has not met with immense popularity. Several reasons may account for this. Despite its logic, converting one's home equity remains a novel idea for many. Some older people loathe the idea of going into debt in their later years. Others are concerned about reducing the size of their estate for their heirs. It is also possible that the additional income may make some of them ineligible for certain government programs.

An explicit form of saving for retirement is the Individual Retirement Account (IRA). It was authorized in the Employee Retirement Income Security Act (ERISA) of 1974. Effective beginning in 1975, an IRA is a tax-deductible and tax-deferred individual savings mechanism available through financial institutions such as commercial banks, saving and loan associations, mutual savings banks, mutual funds, life insurance companies, brokerage houses, and credit unions. The current law (since 1986) permits anyone under age 70¹/₂ to contribute to an IRA account a maximum of $2,000 per year from employment or self-employment income. A person with a nonworking spouse may establish two IRAs with a combined maximum of $2,250. When both spouses work, they may have two IRAs with a maximum of $2,000 each per year. The federal income tax normally payable on the income placed into IRAs is tax-deferred through a tax deduction; the interest income produced by IRAs is not subject to income tax as it accrues and is also tax-deferred. At age 59¹/₂, one may begin withdrawing from an IRA in either a lump sum or annual installments. All withdrawals, including interest earned, are taxed as ordinary income.

Since 1975, both the number of persons establishing IRAs and the amount of dollars saved have grown, in part owing to a 1981 law permitting workers with pension plans as well as workers without them to open IRAs. The popularity of IRAs results largely, however, from tax deductibility and tax deferral. The higher the income level of the IRA holder, the larger the tax saving is at the time of contributing because of tax deductibility for payments into IRAs under the graduate or progressive system of tax brackets. Therefore, the proportion of persons utilizing IRAs increases as income rises.

IRAs were created to provide a tax incentive for generating additional retirement income to supplement Social Security and private pension benefits. Although IRAs had been rather popular, the Tax Reform Act of 1986, imposing restrictions on their use, dampened the interest in, and reduced the use of, this savings vehicle for retirement.

Employment Income

Employment as a source of income for the elderly has clearly declined over the past three decades. Although 36% of the older population had earnings in 1962, only 21% of them did in 1994. Earnings represented 28% of total income of all older persons in 1962, but accounted for only 18% of their total income in 1994 (Grad, 1996).

Earnings may contribute less to the total income of future older people if their participation in the labor force continues to decline and if the early retirement trend continues. However, it is also possible that earnings may become a more important income source if the elderly remain in the work force longer as a means of enhancing their income position during inflationary times. In addition, if the health status of older persons improves with the decline in the mortality rate, then they may wish to work longer. Finally, low birth rates in recent years and the low rates projected for the future will result in a smaller future labor force (as defined by conventional ages). The elderly may well be called on to stay in the labor force longer. Whether older people would continue as labor force participants depends both on personal circumstances and on a number of societal factors affecting the supply of, and demand for, older workers.

The preceding review of income sources suggests that, under existing institutional arrangements and people's behavioral responses to them, much uncertainty surrounds private pensions, individual savings, and employment as major contributors to the income of elders. Because of the singularly important role of Social Security, attention is now turned to its long-range financial problem.

Reasons for Social Security's Financial Problems

Four major factors seem to account for the rising cost of Social Security. The first two—the growth rate of the population and of the economy—relate to the workings of a traditional pay-as-you-go approach to social insurance programs—an intergenerational transfer model, in which the working generation finances benefits for the retired generation. This system works well as long as the population and the economy are growing sufficiently so that, over the long run, the taxes paid by workers and their employers rise faster than, or at least keep pace with, benefits paid out. In many countries, however, Social Security has become a focus of intense criticism and debate because of sluggish economic growth coupled with population aging.

A third factor in Social Security's escalating costs is the eternal temptation of politicians to promise ever-increasing types and levels of benefits. Finally, there is the historical fact that many social programs, including Social Security, are begun when economic and/or demographic conditions are favorable, without regard for the long run. Over time, as economic and demographic conditions change, an imbalance between the program's income and what it spends can develop. If government fails to act or acts too slowly to correct the imbalance, the program deteriorates.

Privatization of Social Security   Solution ①

Many ideas exist for reforming Social Security and one approach is privatization. Privatization of Social Security means that the primary responsibility for retirement income would shift from the taxpayer and government to workers who would be required to save and to invest these savings in the private sector. Are individuals in general able and eager to manage their own investments? What opportunity cost will be incurred if they must do so? If, instead, money-managers do it for them, how much will such services cost? What should the role of society be in cases of investment failure?

The privatization debate essentially revolves around the advantages and disadvantages of defined benefit plans with pay-as-you-go financing, as compared to defined contribution plans. In general, Social Security is a defined benefit plan; it guarantees a benefit based on a predetermined formula. Privatized plans are defined contribution plans; they do *not* guarantee a specified level of retirement income. Under defined contribution plans, the worker, alone or with his or her employer, accumulates savings over time. The level of income during retirement depends on the amount saved and the preretirement investment earnings, taking into account actuarial and financial circumstances at retirement when the total accumulation is converted into a legal contract for income payments. This issue is obviously important because it concerns the adequacy of retirement income.

Most advocates of privatizing Social Security assume that the interest rates earned by the investable funds will be high. However, the financial market, like all other markets, has two sides—supply and demand. Increasing savings will increase the supply of investable funds. Unless the demand for investable funds increases commensurately, market forces will lower the rate of interest. While rates of investment return may be high for some periods of time in a country where privatization is implemented, it cannot be assumed that the rates of return will be consistently high over the long run.

Social Security generally provides retirement, survivorship, and disability benefits in a single package. No private insurance carrier offers an equivalent policy. Typically, advocates of privatization point to higher retirement benefits that they contend could be offered by private investments. They are generally silent, however, about the benefits for survivors and for the disabled. Some proponents for privatization do try to provide for survivorship benefits and disability benefits with a life insurance policy and disability income policy. But they frequently illustrate the costs for providing these benefits by quoting the premiums private insurance carriers charge for those policies, which are lower due to their underwriting requirements. Moreover, not all occupations are insurable for disability by private insurance, and among those that are insurable, premiums for the same benefits can differ considerably by occupational category.

In addition, when part or all of the taxes that go into Social Security are converted into private investments, privatization's effects on income redistribution must be recognized. Under Social Security, low-income earners receive benefits that are proportionately larger than the taxes they have paid into the program compared to higher income earners. This feature of social adequacy under Social Security (i.e., the transfer to low-income earners) will be reduced or eliminated. Moreover, under privatization, investment returns determine the level of retirement income. Those who invest unwisely or are simply unlucky will receive uncertain and meager amounts of income. Unless society can tolerate some of its citizens living in squalor or destitution, the cost of welfare for people who have not been able to save enough or who have failed in their investments must be paid. This income redistribution will be principally from higher-income people, through the first pillar (taxation), thus reducing the higher returns which the well-to-do are expected to receive through the second or third pillar (savings or investments).

Finally, a serious question about the transition remains. How do we move from the current system of Social Security to a world envisioned by the privatizers? Because Social Security is financed on an essentially pay-as-you-go basis under which current taxes are used to pay current benefits, how are benefits to be paid when some or all of the taxes are redirected to privatized accounts? The costs involved in the transition to the new system need to be paid. Are workers now and those in the foreseeable future expected to (1) help pay for the benefits promised to current beneficiaries and those in the transition period and (2) contribute to the privatized accounts for their own retirements?

Redesigning Social Security   Solutions 2,3,4

The way to rectify Social Security's problem is not to dismantle it and to replace it with a privatized plan, as some have proposed. There is nothing intrinsically wrong with the social insurance model. Practically all of its financial problems have resulted from poor plan design and unwise policy decisions in the face of a slowing economy and an aging population. A better policy choice would be to redesign Social Security, making it as self-adjusting and self-sustaining as possible. A sustainable policy is one that adapts automatically to changing conditions. By its very design, an adaptable program prevents hidden time bombs from developing in the first place.

How may the Social Security program be redesigned to deal with the economic and demographic causes of its financial problems? Discussed here are three most useful components in a redesigned program: A wage-based system, a formula-based normal retirement age, and gradual retirement with partial pension.

A WAGE-BASED SYSTEM.[1] A major economic cause of the program's financial instability arises from the fact that its income depends on the payroll tax, which is based on wages, and its outgo reflects prices of goods and services, which determine the cost-of-living adjustments. The difference between the annual rate of change in the average wage and the annual rate of change in the Consumer Price Index (CPI) is known as the real-wage differential. Variations in this differential can have a major impact on costs of the Social Security system.

The benefit structure can be made more nearly self-sustaining if the law provides that the automatic benefit increases will be based on the increase in the nationwide average wage rate minus some fixed percentage point (National Commission on Social Security Reform, 1982). The fixed percentage point should be chosen according to what the real-wage differential is expected to be over the long run. This procedure will result in a benefit computation based solely on one element—wages—thereby eliminating the instability brought about by the wage level and the price level changing at rates that diverge from those assumed in the actuarial model.

Basing Social Security's income and its outgo on wages would substantially stabilize its financing position insofar as variations in economic conditions pertaining to wages and prices are concerned. Aside from providing financial stability, a wage-based system will improve the relative equity between workers and retirees. Thus, if economic conditions are very favorable, beneficiaries would see their benefits increase, reflecting some of the general increase in the standard of living based on wage increases, which will exceed the CPI growth. Conversely, if economic conditions are unfavorable, benefit increases will be less than rises in the CPI so that beneficiaries would share in the general misfortune of the working population.

This proposal would not solve any financial problems arising from other economic elements, such as the unemployment rate. Nonetheless, the real-wage differential is by far the most important economic element in the long-range financing of the Social Security program (National Commission on Social Security Reform, 1982).

A FORMULA-BASED NORMAL RETIREMENT AGE.[2] The demographic cause of Social Security's financial problems results from the demographic load, that is, the ratio of beneficiaries to workers/taxpayers. The U.S. demographic load is projected to increase by 58% by the year 2030. To prevent Social Security costs as a percentage of taxable payroll from increasing significantly will require addressing the rapid growth in the number of beneficiaries relative to the number of workers. Raising the normal retirement age is one way to moderate the rise in total benefit payments.

One way to reset the normal retirement age is to keep constant the ratio between (a) retirement-life expectancy and (b) potential working life (Bayo and Faber, 1981; Chen, 1987). The former refers to the average expected years of life at the normal retirement age. The latter is defined by the number of years between age 20 and the normal retirement age. Suppose the ratio between (a) and (b) is 1 to 3 in year x (e.g., 1940). Assume that the average retirement-life expectancy increases by one year by a future year y (e.g., 1990). If the ratio between (a) and (b) is kept constant (the same in both years), then a one-year extension of life will result in an increase of roughly 3 months of retirement and roughly 9 months of work in year y.

However, increasing the normal retirement age is a contentious issue and ignites spirited debate. To avoid the inaction that often comes with such controversy, it might be preferable to reset the normal retirement age periodically (say, once every 10 years) on an automatic basis according to national statistics on average life expectancy at the current normal retirement age. If an automatic extension of the normal retirement age can be part of the law, then the cost of Social Security attributable to increasing longevity could be systematically controlled.

GRADUAL RETIREMENT WITH PARTIAL PENSIONS. A third element in the redesign of the program is to institute a system of partial pensions for partial retirement, thus coordinating the policy on Social Security with the policy on older-worker employment. At present, workers who want to retire gradually with an interim period of part-time employment confront a number of obstacles. Occupational pension plans rarely allow a beneficiary to continue working for the same firm. If a beneficiary finds employment, Social Security lowers benefits for those who earn beyond an allowable amount through the earnings test—a considerable work disincentive to persons with earnings beyond the annual exempt amount.

People work for a variety of reasons, and these reasons change as workers grow older. Many say that they are willing and able to work longer than they currently do, especially on a part-time basis. At age 63 and over, for example, "enjoying work" is the most frequently cited reason for working, followed by feeling useful, being productive, regarding work as an obligation, and maintaining health insurance. Significantly, the need for income is mentioned least often (U.S. Department of Labor, 1989).

Slow economic growth and population aging have raised concerns about the ability of society to finance pensions (public and private) and health services for the elderly. In addition, projections of a slower growth in the working-age population have led to concerns about labor force shortages in the future. One way to mitigate these problems is to prolong the working life of older people. Postponing the normal retirement age, coupled with a desire on the part of older people to work part-time (as expressed in practice and in opinion surveys) would seem to provide a recipe for gradual retirement. Partial pensions for partial retirement may be a practicable approach.

In order to implement gradual retirement with partial pensions, institutional and attitudinal changes are needed. If we assume the willingness of older workers to remain in the labor market, occupational pension and Social Security provisions that offer retirement incentives (or work disincentives) should be eliminated. For example, the delayed retirement credit under Social Security should be made actuarially fair immediately, not waiting until the year 2009 as provided under current law.[3] In order to accommodate workers in general and older workers in particular, flexible work schedules and training/retraining programs should be more widely and systematically available. The types of available jobs are also important. If, indeed, part-time jobs are what are needed to implement partial pensions, then the willingness of employers to create such opportunities and the cooperation of full-time workers to support them will be necessary.

To promote gradual retirement by means of partial pensions would require a major change in Social Security and occupational pension programs. However, to implement gradual retirement in the United States through a system of part-time work with partial pensions will have many salubrious effects, including easing the concern over the extension of the normal retirement age.

Conclusion

This chapter reviewed the relative roles and present status of various sources from which the elderly receive income: Social Security, private pensions, assets, and employment. From historical and current statistics, it is evident that Social Security is the most significant source of income—in 1994, 91% of elders received Social Security and it accounted for 42% of all the income they received.

Because of the enduring importance of Social Security, the chapter then discusses the long-range actuarial deficit under the program that was highlighted, pointing out the root causes of its financial problem, analyzing the issues surrounding privatization, and arguing for creating a self-sustaining and financially stable Social Security.

With a stable Social Security program as a foundation for a basic level of retirement income, other means of income support, including a privatized system of saving and investment, can then be used as supplements to ensure income security.

With income security, attention should then be turned to a more comprehensive concern about economic security. Mechanisms

for providing health care should always be included when addressing economic security since the latter is a broader concept than
income security, concerning not only the acquisition of income and
assets, but also the retention and disposal of income. It is well-
known, for example, that the elderly when compared to the
nonelderly are at greater risk and must budget more for medical
and personal care services. Potentially significant expenditures for
health care, however, generally are not given explicit consideration
in assessments of the economic status of the elderly versus the
nonelderly.

A more accurate assessment of economic security, therefore,
may be accomplished only when income, accumulated wealth, and
consumption expenditures are comprehensively considered from the
standpoint of supply and demand. In that light, income and wealth
represent the supply of resources, and consumption represents the
demand on those resources. For example, even if the elderly have
achieved income and wealth levels on a par with those of the
nonelderly—their command over resources being equal, it does not
follow that their economic security is the same as younger groups,
because older people are faced with an actual or a potential higher
demand on resources for health care, including long term care (see
chapter by Binstock in this volume). In short, the importance of
health care and long-term care to the older population cannot be
overemphasized.

Notes

1. Some may feel that this discussion neglects to address the inequities in earnings and work histories for women and minorities. There
ought not to be such a concern, however, since the proposed procedure only
affects the computation for automatic benefit increases.

2. Some may be concerned about the distributional implications for
minorities arising from their differences in mortality and disability. Postponing normal retirement age should in principle not affect disability
benefits. It does, however, have differential effects on those with shorter
life expectancies and those without continued employment (beyond the
previously set normal retirement age). The gradual retirement proposal,
discussed in the next section, would deal with the impact of normal retirement age postponement, since it would enable people to receive retirement
benefits sooner in the form of partial pensions.

3. The delayed retirement credit (DRC) is designed to compensate
workers for not receiving benefits when they defer retirement. In other

words, the DRC increases their future benefits. The DRC rate, under existing law, is 4.5% for persons born in 1929 or 1930. This is scheduled to rise to 8% for those born in 1943 or later. When the DRC is at the rate of 8%, the compensation will become actuarially fair, in the sense that what one does not receive today, one will receive tomorrow. However, for all those born before 1943, thus attaining the normal retirement age before the year 2009, the compensation is actuarially unfair, because future increases in benefits are less in present value terms than the current reductions in benefits.

References

Bayo, F. R., and Faber, J. (1981). Equivalent retirement ages: 1940–2050 (Actuarial Note no. 105).

Chen, Y. P. (1987). Making assets out of tomorrow's elderly. *The Gerontologist*, 27, 410–16.

———. (1995a). Home equity conversion. In G. L. Maddox (Ed.), *The Encyclopedia of Aging*, 2d ed., pp. 426–63. New York: Springer Publishing.

———. (1995b). Income security a key concern for elders. *Aging Today*, January/February, 7, 10.

Grad, S. (1996). *Income of the population 55 or older, 1992*. Washington, DC: Social Security Admministration Publication no. 13–11871.

OASDI Board of Trustees. (1996). 1996 annual report of the Federal Old-Age and Survivors Insurance and Disability Insurance Trust Funds. Washington, DC: U.S. Government Printing Office.

National Commission on Social Security Reform (1982). Staff Memoranda nos. 16, 19, and 26.

Radner, D. B. (1988). *The wealth of the aged and nonaged, 1984*. Office of Research and Statistics Working Paper Series, no. 36. Washington, DC: Social Security Administration.

U.S. Department of Labor. (1989). *Older worker task force: Key police issues for the future*. Report to the Secretary of Labor. Washington, DC: U.S. Government Printing Office.

Chapter 4

Housing and Supportive Services for the Elderly: Intergenerational Perspectives and Options

PHOEBE S. LIEBIG

During the 1960s and 1970s, the dominant rubric of age-based policy centered on the needs of the elderly, who were described as poor and suffering from multiple losses—to be old was to be in need. More recently, a new stereotype of well-off "Greedy Geezers" has emerged, thereby obscuring the heterogeneity of those aged 65 and over. A growing body of knowledge about aging has identified numerous differences among the elderly, with a need to create policies sensitive to these distinctions (Bass, Kutza, and Torres-Gil, 1990). This *intragenerational* diversity requires greater scrutiny if we are to develop more adequate policies for the twenty-first century, when one of every five Americans will be aged 65 and older.

This chapter addresses the issue of affordable and suitable housing for the elderly, first by examining some intragroup differences among the elderly, especially their housing status. Next, federal and state policies that have helped shape this status are examined, as are various housing options available to different groups of elders. A final section discusses future housing policy suggesting that housing inequality among the aged will persist in the next century, partly driven by today's political climate.

Intragroup Differences among the Elderly

Differences among the elderly have important impacts on their housing needs. First, the older population is aging. In the mid-1990s,

51

persons aged 65 and older numbered 33.2 million or 12.7% of the total U.S. population; 2.8% of all Americans were aged 80 and over, the group most likely to be physically and mentally frail. By the year 2025, there will be 59.7 million elders; 4.6% will be aged 80 and older (U.S. Congress, 1991). Most of these "oldest-old" will be women living alone who need supportive services to remain in their own homes.

The elderly are also becoming more racially and ethnically diverse (Torres-Gil, 1992). In 1990, 28.3 million elderly were white; 2.6 million were Black; 1.1 million were Hispanic; and .6 million were other groups, such as Native Americans and Asians (see chapter by Villa in this volume). Of the projected 69 million persons aged 65 and older in the year 2050, 10 million will be Black, 8 million will be Hispanic, and 5 million from other races (Taeuber, 1992). Many are and will be ill-housed.

The older population is not distributed uniformly among the fifty states, with important implications for state-level housing and long-term care policies. The majority are clustered in nine states: California in the West; Florida and Texas in the South; New York, New Jersey, and Pennsylvania in the East; and Ohio, Illinois, and Michigan in the Midwest (American Association of Retired Persons [AARP], 1994). Eight Western states have experienced the largest increases since 1990 in the proportion of state population aged 65 and older; Nevada leads with a 22% jump over the past four years. Higher proportions (more than 20%) of poor elderly live in eight southern states with large rural and minority populations; Mississippi has the greatest proportion of elders (29.3%) living in poverty (AARP, 1994).

Income differences by virtue of age and gender are especially pronounced. Elders aged 85 and over have higher rates of poverty (18.5%) than all the elderly (12.8%). In 1990, the median family unit income for aged 85 and older was $11,728 or 63% of the median family unit income for aged 65 to 69. Younger old men (aged 65–69) had incomes of $20,260 compared to $13,520 for men over age 85. Women fared less well, with the younger old having incomes of $17,246, compared to those over age 85 with $10,468. Oldest-old women living alone were the worst off, with incomes of $8,120 (Radner, 1993).

Median household wealth also differs by age. In 1990, the net worth of aged 65 to 69 households was $59,128 compared to $47,599 for households aged 80 and over (Radner, 1993). Similar to younger persons, the greatest asset of the elderly is their home.

Home equity represents 42% of household net worth of persons over age 80; for the oldest women living alone, it is 52% (ibid.).

The health status of the older population also varies. Poorer individuals are less healthy; 40% of elders with annual incomes below $10,000 (a group dominated by aged 75 and over) rate their health as fair or poor (U.S. Congress, 1991). Similarly, health care expenditures vary by income and age (see chapter by Binstock in this volume). For example, in 1989, the "young old" (aged 65–74) spent an average of $1,981 out-of-pocket on health care, in contrast with the $2,351 spent by those aged 75 and over (U.S. Congress, 1991).

Many elderly also incur expenses for nonmedical assistance that enables them to stay in their apartments and houses. This includes help with shopping, transportation, and other instrumental activities of daily living (IADLs). Disabled elders, particularly the oldest-old or those suffering from Alzheimer's disease or from other cognitive impairments, may also require help with bathing, feeding, and other activities of daily living (ADLs). Many families perform these tasks but formal paid assistance may also be needed.

From the foregoing, it is clear that today's older adults in their eighth and ninth decades and beyond, especially minorities, fit the stereotype attributed to all elderly in the 1960s and 1970s. They are more likely to be poor, increasingly frail, and needing assistance provided in their homes.

Housing Profile of the Elderly

These intragroup differences are reflected in the housing status of the elderly, best described by tenure (i.e., whether people own or rent) and expenditure patterns. In 1991, nearly one-fourth of all U.S.-owned or -rented homes included an elderly person. Of those more than 20 million households, 13 million were single-person households; 8.8 million were headed by a person aged 75 and over. Renter-occupied older households numbered 4.6 million, with a median age of 75 and over. Approximately 70% of older renters, predominantly women, were persons living alone (U.S. Department of Commerce and U.S. Department of Housing and Urban Development, 1993).

The elderly have high rates of homeownership. In 1993, 77% of all the elderly were homeowners (AARP, 1994). These rates are described by an inverted U-shaped curve, peaking among those in their early 60s and falling with advanced age. This reflects the fact that many of today's oldest households never became homeowners due to the depression, especially women who never married. By contrast, somewhat younger elders who were part of the post-World War II "marriage boom" became homeowners, benefiting from various government policies, including the GI Bill (Pynoos and Redfoot, 1995). The drop in oldest-old ownership also reflects a pattern of moving into apartments that are easier to maintain.

From 1980 to 1987, the rate of homeownership among the young old (aged 65–74) increased from 77% to 81%, the largest increase for any age group; for those aged 75 and over, the increase was less than 1% (Mikleson and Turner, 1990). Homeownership among the elderly, however, is not a function of affluence; 60% of all older households with annual incomes under $5,000 are homeowners. Because older persons tend to be reluctant to move, preferring to "age in place," a majority live in homes where the mortgage is fully paid or almost so. Nearly 60% own homes free of any mortgage obligation (Cook and Settersen, 1995).

These older homes, however, are often unsuitable because they need major maintenance and repair or environmental modifications to enable their older residents to function more independently and safely. Approximately one million elders could benefit from home modifications that promote self-care or the delivery of care by informal and formal caregivers (Struyk and Katsura, 1987).

Poor quality housing is concentrated among poor, rural, and minority elders and those living alone (Pynoos and Redfoot, 1995; Redfoot and Gaberlavage, 1991). More than 6% of older persons live in homes needing structural repair and maintenance; 11.4% of rural elders need this service. As expected, income and housing adequacy are closely related. Only 4.4% of elderly households with incomes between $10,000 and $15,000 live in severely inadequate housing, contrasted with nearly 9% of elder households with incomes between $5,000 and $10,000. Fully 17.4% of those with incomes below $5,000 have inadequate housing. Only 4% of white elders, but 12.5% of Hispanic and 23% of Black elderly homeowners live in moderately to severely inadequate housing. Golant and LaGreca (1994) suggest that certain longtime homeowners, such as the very poor, Blacks, and men living alone, are less able to maintain their homes and may have significant dwelling deficiencies.

Housing adequacy is especially a problem for older renters. Nearly 6% of white renters have inadequate housing, as do 16.6% of elderly Hispanics and 21.2% of older Blacks (Golant and LaGreca,

1994). For both owners and renters, home repair programs can raise the quality of housing, while home modifications (e.g., grab bars) can provide a more supportive and safer environment.

During the period between 1980 and 1987, older renters became significantly older and poorer. Renters aged 65 to 74 declined by 2%; those aged 75 and over increased by 20%. Older renters with incomes of less than $5,000 grew astronomically—by 63%; conversely, the numbers of elder renters with incomes of $25,000 or greater declined by 25% (Mikleson and Turner, 1990; Pynoos and Redfoot, 1995).

Older renters pay more of their income for housing than older homeowners. In 1987, 60% of renters aged 65 to 74 and 66% of renters aged 75 and over had excessive housing costs. By contrast, 16% of owners aged 65 to 74 and 17% of owners aged 75 and over had excessive costs, defined by the Department of Housing and Urban Development (HUD) in this case as more than 40% of income (Mikleson and Turner, 1990).

Housing and housing-related expenditures made by the elderly have continued to be higher than health care expenditures, a spending pattern similar to that of the nonelderly. In 1991, more than 30% of elder households paid more than 30% of their income on housing, the current federal standard for excessive rent (U.S. Department of Commerce and U.S. Department of Housing and Urban Development, 1993). Even more telling is the proportion of total income spent on housing by the aged. Those over age 75 spend more on housing, ranging from 38.4% of income in the highest quintile, to 44.9% in the lowest income group. For the young old, the range is from 31.6% in the highest quintile to 38.7% in the lowest (Cook and Settersen, 1995).

The housing status of today's elders can be summarized in the following fashion. Older Americans are predominantly homeowners, even those with very low incomes, but homeownership is higher among the young-old. Housing costs constitute nearly one-fourth of all older persons' expenditures; more than 30% of the elderly pay more than the federal standard for excessive rent. This expenditure pattern is especially prevalent among renters over aged 75, who are primarily women. The cost of housing for American elders limits available choices, especially for the low-income aged and the oldest-old. Poor quality housing is a problem, especially for those who live in rural areas, have very low incomes, and/or are Hispanic, Black, women, or renters. These intragroup differences have been shaped, in part, by federal and state housing policies.

Housing Policies

Modern U.S. housing policy mirrors that of other Western industrialized nations; before 1900, governments took almost no direct responsibility for housing. Two world wars and a global economic depression eroded this stance against public sector involvement. Post-World War II trends, such as increased marriage rates and larger proportions of the elderly, led to an expanded role for the U.S. national government. Housing programs became intimately tied to national economic policy and to the financial security of households (Heidenheimer, Heclo, and Adams, 1983).

Federal Housing Policy

While U.S. housing policy has centered on maintaining a strong private housing market aided by the national government, the states and localities also play an important role, as does (to a lesser degree) the nonprofit housing sector. Our housing policy has been guided by a supplementary, rather than a comprehensive approach, with a focus on those groups unable to secure housing in the private market (e.g., the poor and the elderly). It consists primarily of a (1) mortgage-guarantee program, coupled with substantial tax preferences for homeownership; and (2) a relatively modest subsidy program of federally assisted housing production and rental assistance.

The elderly have been major beneficiaries of both programs, with high rates of homeownership, as just noted, and a dominant share of occupancy in the limited amount of public and subsidized housing (Pynoos and Liebig, 1995). For example, of very low-income households receiving federal rent subsidies, nearly one-fourth are elderly; 45% of the 1.2 million public housing units are occupied by the elderly (Turner, 1989). The aged also have benefited from home rehabilitation or weatherization programs for low-income households.

Besides being major recipients of programs designed for low-income households (e.g., Section 8 rental assistance, enacted in 1974 so that only 30% of income is paid for rent), elders also have benefited from age-specific housing policies since 1959. Over the years, the Section 202 rental housing construction program has subsidized nonprofit sponsors to develop nearly 300,000 rental units for ambulatory moderate- and low-income elders ineligible for public housing. Approximately 10% of the units were made accessible for disabled persons, but services were not guaranteed. Residents or sponsors were responsible for meal programs and other services, with the Older Americans Act (OAA) and state funds used to fill service gaps. In 1974 the Section 202 program was retargeted to low-income elderly and linked to Section 8 rental assistance.

During the late 1960s and early 1970s, there was a growing recognition that "suitable" housing for the elderly encompassed more than a "bricks and mortar" approach of producing affordable housing (Pynoos and Liebig, 1995). A demonstration program to combine services with housing—the Congregate Housing Services Program (CHSP)—was initiated in 1978. The CHSP was designed to offer a service-rich setting for elders who had "aged in place" and who become frail over time in federally subsidized housing. HUD was to ensure the availability of services, a task seen by some staff as outside their normal role of housing production.

A similar demonstration program in rural areas was implemented from 1979 to 1983 by the Farmers Home Administration (FmHA), in cooperation with the Administration on Aging. It consisted of earmarked loans for rental construction, assistance funds, and a minimum package of supportive services managed by a service coordinator. By 1988, the FmHA had made 47 loans to build or renovate housing, accounting for about 600 units nationwide (Struyk et al., 1989). Despite attempts by the Reagan administration to zero out the CHSP and to reduce the Section 202 program, Congress continued to fund the former. The Reagan administration, however, was successful in severely curtailing the overall federal housing role in the 1980s (Pynoos and Redfoot, 1995).

A more proactive role was signaled by the bipartisan passage of the National Affordable Housing Act (NAHA) in 1990. Included were programs targeted to the elderly, as well as several nonage-specific programs affecting elders' housing, such as the Community Development Block Grant (CDBG) program. A revised Section 202 put more emphasis on supportive services and financed the construction and rehabilitation of any structure to be used for supportive housing for very low-income elders, through capital advances and contracts for rental assistance. Funding for on-site service coordinators also was included as an eligible cost.

The NAHA authorized up to $51 million over a two-year period for a revised CHSP to cover services and retrofitting of individual dwelling units and public and common spaces to accommodate the special needs of frail older and younger disabled persons. A new demonstration program, HOPE for Elderly Independence, was initiated to test the effectiveness of combining housing vouchers with supportive services to help 1,500 elders live independently. Both the revised CHSP and HOPE program required cost sharing: 50% from the sponsoring agency, 40% from federal funds, and 10% from client fees. This same formula was required for the HOME program to fund new construction, moderate and substantial rehabilitation of existing buildings, and tenant-based assistance. These cost-sharing requirements came at a difficult time for states and localities with budgetary problems. One consequence was that only about half of the localities expected to submit the required planning document did so (Hoban and Richardson, 1992).

In addition, the NAHA authorized an expansion of the Home Equity Conversion Mortgage (HECM) demonstration program from 5,000 to 25,000 contracts. First introduced in Maine in 1961, HECMs became a national program in 1987. They allow older persons to convert the equity in their homes to a monthly income, without having to relocate. The expanded program was undergirded by federal insurance to protect borrowers and lenders and the willingness of the Federal National Mortgage Association ("Fannie Mae") to provide a secondary mortgage market for lenders and to market the program to consumers.

Any person aged 62 or older, with a home in good condition that is the principal residence and free and clear of a mortgage, is eligible for this program. The owner must receive counseling from a HUD-approved agency. Early research showed that more than one-third of near poor elders could receive at least $2,000 annually for the rest of their lives (Jacobs and Weissert, 1984). The very poor, however, are less likely to benefit; the value of their homes is often insufficient for lenders to assume such a long-range risk.

A recent report on the program (Barriere, 1992) revealed that the average age of all participants was 77. A relatively small number of loans (1,703) was made between November 1989 and June 1992. The average value of the properties involved was $128,000; the average income of participants was just slightly over $7,500 annually, 94% derived from Social Security. Participants were primarily nonminority (95.6% white), predominantly females living alone (56%) and secondarily, males living with others (29%). While lenders were active in the District of Columbia and thirty-two states, the five most active states were California, New York, Rhode Island, New Jersey, and Colorado (Barriere, 1992).

Recent Political Environment

The 1992 reauthorization of the NAHA, the Housing and Community Development Act, embodied many of the provisions of the

1990 act. Mortgage insurance for the production of assisted living facilities was added. The Clinton administration attempted to reduce the number of new Section 202 units and the CHSP program, but Congress reinstated them. The 1994 reauthorization, however, encountered more severe difficulties and after the November 1994 elections these problems were compounded by a consistently partisan environment.

The Clinton administration proposed in its American Community Partnerships Act a series of "performance-based" housing grants, which closely resemble block grants. In keeping with the climate of providing greater discretion to the states, few mandates would be operative, such as requiring age-specific programs. One possible outcome is a reduction in the linking of housing and services for the approximately one million frail low- and moderate-income elderly residents in government-assisted housing. The administration's proposed reauthorization in 1995 of the Older Americans Act, a modest but important funding source for services, also proposed greater discretion to the states and localities. Individuals not residing in government-assisted housing may have a higher priority in state and local allocations of these limited funds.

Since the new Republican majority took charge in the House, rescissions of existing budgets and proposed cuts in programs have dominated the housing agenda. The CHSP suffered in the FY95 budget rescissions, as did the Low-Income Home Energy Assistance Program (LIHEAP), both important programs for low-income elders. The House proposed a 27% reduction in HUD FY96 funding from FY95 levels and a new "Special Needs Housing" fund to consolidate funding for Section 202 and for housing for persons with disabilities and with AIDS, not dissimilar from the president's housing proposals. HUD funding was finally enacted via a full-year continuing resolution more than six months after the start of FY96. Less than a month later, the House passed the U.S. Housing Act of 1996, which would go even further in reducing the national role by repealing the Housing Act of 1937 and devolving a significant amount of authority to local agencies. Should the Senate enact similar legislation, the federal role may be reduced substantially, as it was in the 1980s, with greater devolution to the states and localities, accompanied by fewer federal dollars.

State Housing Policy

Housing for older Americans has traditionally been a state policy objective (Schwartz, Ferlauto, and Hoffman, 1988). Until the

early 1980s, state-level public policies in elderly housing were,
however, largely derived from federal policies (Schwartz, 1984).
The largest single activity in almost every state was the utilization
of federal authority to issue tax-free housing bonds and federal
rent subsidies to produce dwelling units for income- or asset-eligible
elders. With the passage of the Tax Reform Act of 1986 that eliminated many tax advantages for developers, all states allocated some
tax credits for construction of low- and moderate-income housing.
By the mid-1980s, eight states had provided tax-exempt bond
financing for the construction of congregate housing facilities. Twenty
percent of the units were reserved for low-income elderly tenants;
providing supportive services was the developer's responsibility
(Struyk et al., 1989).

These federal tax policy changes and the federal government
withdrawal in the 1980s from a proactive role in public and subsidized housing production and a shift to tenant-based assistance
(e.g., housing vouchers) led to other state action. Despite recessionary
pressures, the states moved away from their historical role of serving largely as conduits for federal subsidies. Many states used their
own tax revenues to fund existing housing and to create new housing and supportive housing programs. More than a hundred new
programs were created in forty states, the majority of them in
Connecticut, Massachusetts, and Maryland (Turner, 1989).

Many of these programs were focused on developing *supportive housing*, that is, the integration of housing with a range
of services (e.g., meals, laundry, and personal care) to semi-
independent, low-income elders with functional impairments who
require assistance with IADLs and ADLs, but not the skilled nursing care provided in nursing homes. The most popular approach
was to subsidize a specified core of supportive services, funded by
state appropriations, the OAA, Medicaid, and Social Services Block
Grant (SSBG) funds. The differing funding streams and eligibility
requirements for different programs, however, often made it difficult
to create adequate service packages and required higher levels of
interagency coordination between the state departments or bureaus
administering these several programs. A survey of State Units on
Aging (SUAs) found that, despite the OAA mandate to develop a
comprehensive system of community- and home-based care, SUA
interactions with their state housing finance agencies or housing
and community development departments were infrequent (Liebig,
1995). In addition, despite the NAHA requirements for a bottom-up
planning mechanism, the Comprehensive Housing Affordability

Strategy (CHAS) that included consultation with social services agencies such as the SUAs, only thirty-five state aging agencies participated in that process by early 1993 (Liebig, 1994).

Another state policy initiative in the 1980s consisted of creating a statewide human service coordinator to provide technical assistance and resource information to managers of government-assisted housing with low-income elderly tenants. While no new services were established, local health and social service resources were assessed and training provided for managers and prospective developers concerning the service needs of elderly residents. Only a few states developed this model; instead, two other approaches were utilized. In one, the housing manager assessed tenant needs and arranged for services; in the other, additional staff were hired to assist tenants and arrange for services (Struyk et al., 1989). The latter approach was the precursor of the on-site coordinator featured in NAHA.

Other state-level supportive housing initiatives, on a less widespread basis, included the retrofitting of existing buildings (e.g., motels, convents, and schools) to accommodate housing with services and the creation of computer software or housing directories to provide information on available housing options statewide. One program, inaugurated by the Robert Wood Johnson Foundation (RWJ) in 1988, sought to test a model of developing services for the vast numbers of tenants who reside in apartments that are not public housing. The Supportive Services Program in Senior Housing (SSPSH) provided three-year funding to ten state housing finance agencies (HFAs) to integrate and coordinate agencies and resources through market analysis, service-package design, and training. The beneficiaries of these leveraged efforts were elderly residents of HFA-financed housing developments. In contrast to the CHSP model of highly targeted services, the RWJ program was driven by an emphasis on consumer sovereignty and open to all tenants. An evaluation of the SSPSH revealed that HFAs and sponsors were willing to provide funds for services coordinators and that tenants were willing and able—even those with limited incomes—to pay a portion of the costs for services such as house cleaning and transportation (Feder, Scanlon, and Howard, 1992; Lanspery, 1992).

Other major state housing initiatives included shared housing, property tax relief, and the regulation of residential long-term care facilities. Shared housing—the matching-up of a person seeking housing with another individual with excess housing capacity or the creation of small group homes that offer the potential advantage of companionship and assistance—was promoted by forty-two states. Despite limited funding for administrative costs, slow consumer acceptance, and concerns about program effectiveness, more than four hundred such programs were developed in the 1980s (National Shared Housing Resource Center, 1989). With the erosion of funding sources, some of which were earmarked for these programs, many programs have leveled off or been discontinued.

State tax policies also have important impacts on housing and related expenditures. The property tax generates approximately 75% of county and 50% of municipal tax revenues (Mackey and Carter, 1994). Thus, it is not only important for financing school districts, but also for a host of local services used by the elderly and other age groups. Indeed, the property tax is often the only significant tax that the growing middle-class elderly population pays to support state and local services (Mackey and Carter, 1994). The income tax, an important source of tax revenue in 40 states (10 states have none or a very limited tax), is often accompanied by tax subsidies that eliminate or reduce tax liability for many middle-income elders. Furthermore, the elderly characteristically spend a higher proportion of their income on nontaxable items such as food and medical care, thus lowering their sales tax burden (ibid.).

Two major kinds of property tax relief exist: homestead credits or exemptions and "circuitbreakers" or property tax deferrals. Forty-six states have a homestead program available to at least one class of qualified homeowner, with veterans and the disabled the most common recipients. Most programs were created during the Depression to help taxpayers avoid foreclosure and were generally available to all homeowners.

New Jersey was the first state to develop an exemption targeted to the elderly; today, 24 states have homestead exemptions for seniors only, with 4 states leaving this policy up to the discretion of their local governments. Sixteen require elderly homeowners to meet income criteria, thereby providing tax relief to those on fixed incomes, not to wealthy retirees (Mackey and Carter, 1994). Homestead exemptions reduce property taxes by exempting a certain amount of the home's value from taxation. Usually mandated by state law, the revenue loss must be absorbed by local governments; otherwise the tax burden must be shifted to other property. Only 12 states reimburse localities for this loss. Nine states and the District of Columbia have homestead credit programs that either involve direct rebates to taxpayers or reduce the property tax bill directly (ibid.).

Circuitbreakers prevent property taxes from placing a tax burden overload on taxpayers. Unlike the homestead programs, these state-financed programs are carefully targeted to low- and moderate-income taxpayers and can benefit homeowners and renters. Initiated by Wisconsin in 1964, the majority of programs were adopted in the 1970s. A total of 31 states currently have these programs; 29 set a maximum income above which homeowners and renters may not qualify, ranging from $3,750 to $100,000. All states set a maximum benefit amount, ranging from $125 to $2,000. Of the 30 states with circuitbreakers for homeowners, 6 do not provide relief to renters, 4 allow all households to participate without regard to age or disability, and 4 provide more generous benefits for the elderly and disabled (Mackey and Carter, 1994).

Like their homeowner program counterparts, circuitbreakers for renters are targeted to the elderly and disabled. Of the 26 states with such programs, only 7 provide the same benefits to all renters without respect to age. Two states (Alaska and Oregon) provide this relief to renters only, while 5 states offer more generous relief to elders (Mackey and Carter, 1994).

Property tax deferrals are another form of tax relief. These programs allow the elderly and in some case disabled homeowners to put off the payment of taxes to a later date. While this form of tax relief is available in 21 states, 5 states offer these programs at the option of local governments. Fifteen of the 21 states require qualifying homeowners to meet income guidelines, while 6 states and the District of Columbia make the program available to all older homeowners of all incomes (Mackey and Carter, 1994). These deferred taxes become a lien against the value of the home; when it is sold, back taxes plus interest become due. If the homeowner dies, the deferred taxes are paid by the estate. These deferral programs are the most targeted method of alleviating concerns about elderly homeowners losing their homes because they cannot afford taxes. Anecdotal reports, however, reveal that many older homeowners are reluctant to have a lien placed against their home. This appears to parallel their disinclination to participate in the HECM program.

Of these three state property tax relief programs, only one provides relief to elderly renters, the segment of the elderly population most likely to pay excessive costs for housing. Furthermore, unlike older homeowners, renters do not have an asset that can generate an income stream to alleviate the burdens of their housing, health, or other expenses.

A final state policy of increasing importance to elderly housing is the regulation of board and care homes (B&Cs) and assisted living facilities (ALFs). Both state and local governments have increased their regulation of B&Cs that provide a room, meals, help with ADLs, and some degree of protective oversight. All states have laws regulating this form of supportive housing, often with monitoring by multiple agencies, depending on the size and type of facility and populations served. The major focus is on the physical condition and operation of these homes; many standards are similar to those required of nursing homes (see Dobkin, 1989). The service-mix varies widely; in several states, residents of B&Cs are often not provided with OAA-funded services (Hawes, Wildfire, and Lux, 1993). Thus, low- and moderate-income residents may not receive publicly funded services that they would, if they were living in their own homes or with others.

The advent of ALFs, a service-enriched residential environment, often purpose-built (rather than a converted private home, as occurs with B&Cs) and staffed by professionals, has given rise to other residential facility regulation issues. Some of these stem from definitional problems as to whether ALFs are the same or different from B&Cs and therefore, require the same kind of state intervention to protect consumers (Mollica et al., 1992). Middle- and upper-income, frail elders increasingly are targeted by builders of ALFs; this form of supportive housing is becoming more popular among those who can afford it. In some instances, this level of housing and care has been added to existing retirement communities and Continuing Care Retirement Community campuses and also as separate wings or adjacent buildings in skilled nursing facilities (Regnier, Hamilton, and Yatabe, 1991; Regnier, 1994). While these regulatory issues have not become politicized since the Republican takeover of many statehouses since November 1994, they are part of the growing concerns of state policymakers, regardless of party, about long-term care costs.

Housing Options

Since the 1960s federal and state housing policies have sought to meet the housing needs of the elderly, initially with a focus on the provision of affordable housing for both homeowners and renters, and more recently, with an emphasis on combining housing and services for the growing numbers of frail elders. Housing, however, has never been an entitlement. Major efforts have been targeted to increasing and sustaining home ownership among the elderly of all income levels and in all parts of the country, a policy thrust that has largely succeeded. Policies benefiting older renters have fluctuated, with the federal government withdrawing from this arena in the 1980s, and likely to do so again, for the remainder of the 1990s. Older renters are disadvantaged, relative to home-owners, because low-income housing options such as rural and small-town apartment complexes and Single Residency Occupancy hotels and rooming houses in cities are in short supply, relative to the level of need. As noted by Golant (1992), the problem of appropriate housing for American elders has generated a number of possible solutions, but few actual choices.

Table 4.1 describes some of the major housing possibilities that are open to elders. Many are increasingly available to upper-middle- and upper-income suburban elders. This is especially true of supportive housing options, such as ALFs and CCRCs, built by for-profit developers and supported by the secondary mortgage market. With the current political climate driving reductions in federal construction and rental assistance programs for the poor and those targeted to frail elders, such as the CHSP and Section 202 service coordination, lower-income elders will be even more disadvantaged, relative to their higher income counterparts, than in the past. The ability of the states or the nonprofit sector to fill some of these gaps is equivocal. Certainly, the status of subnational government finances, even without the greater possibility of bank-ruptcies such as Orange County in California, raises questions about the ability of states to fund more supportive housing programs for low- and moderate-income elders. Recent state finance studies pro-vide little room for optimism (Snell, 1993).

The Future

Briefly, future intragenerational issues in housing for the eld-erly can be viewed from two perspectives: the short term and the more distant future. In the short term, the likely withdrawal of the federal government from a more proactive role in housing for the elderly does not bode well for the less well-off elderly. This action, coupled with the uneven performance by the states in hous-ing production for the aged and the development of supportive hous-ing, and the private market focus on the types of supportive housing from which a profit can be made, may result in the needs of poorer,

Table 4.1

Housing Options by Location and Income Levels

Type of Option	Location (Metro/Suburban/Exurban/Rural)	Income Levels Served (Very Low to High)
Independent Housing		
Public housing (HUD)	Primarily metropolitan, inner city	Very low to low
Section 202 (HUD)	Primarily metropolitan	Low to moderate
Section 515 (FmHA)	Rural	Very low to low
Single Resident Occupancy hotels (SROs)	Metropolitan (inner city)	Very low to low
Apartments	Metropolitan, suburban, exurban, rural	All, but primarily low
Single-family homes	Metropolitan, suburban, exurban, rural	All
Mobile homes	Suburban, exurban, some rural	Primarily low to moderate
Retirement communities (e.g., Leisure World)	Suburban, exurban	Upper-middle to high
Supportive Housing		
Congregate Housing Services Program (CHSP/HUD)	Sites nationwide	Low to moderate
Section 202 with On-site Service Coordination (Also other federal and state subsidized housing)	Sites nationwide	Low to moderate
Accessory Apartments/ECHO Housing	Suburban, exurban, some rural	Probably moderate
Board and Care	Suburban, exurban, some rural	Low, some moderate
Assisting Living	Primarily suburban, exurban	Upper-middle to high
Continuing Care Retirement Communities (CCRCs)	Primarily suburban, exurban	Upper-middle to high

much older and minority elders being unmet, and even less so than they are today. The economic development motives of the states and their current financial straits may make it less easy to target more resources to disadvantaged elders, whose needs are often not well represented by the mainstream aging interest groups in their advocacy efforts (Day, 1990; Wallace et al., 1991). The prospects for aging interest group influence at the state level also are uncertain; other than AARP and the Alzheimer's Association, most of the gray lobby is not well organized in state capitols (Liebig, 1992). To be successful in Sacramento, Albany, and Boston, aging interest groups may need to focus their advocacy on behalf of middle-class elders.

Other intergovernmental factors also are likely to affect intragenerational issues in housing for the elderly. The extent to which Medicaid becomes more flexible for the states, especially in their ability to funnel those funds to services in small group homes/B&Cs/SROs where poor and low-income elders reside, will have major effects on the supportive housing needs of more needy elders. In addition, the possibility of reduced mandates in the reauthorized OAA, plus the level of funding available, will also have an impact on the types of services and the target groups to be served by that program. Cuts in SSBG funding enacted by the 104th Congress will have a negative impact on the ability of the states to provide in-home services for elders.

Looking ahead to the more distant future, it is likely that intragenerational issues in housing for the elderly will persist. Home ownership among tomorrow's elderly may not be as high as today's. In 1990, home ownership among the nonelderly leveled off at 64%, in contrast to the major jump in American home ownership rates from 44% in 1940 to 55% in 1950, and more gradual increases to 64% in 1980. One somewhat encouraging sign is the near doubling of women-homeowners from 15% in 1940 to 28% in 1990 (Home ownership, 1994)—encouraging, because the ranks of the oldest old will continue to be predominantly female. Having a major asset, such as a home, which can be converted to needed income while providing shelter, will enable the next generations of older women to avoid poverty.

A less positive sign is the continuing reports of greater income inequality in the U.S. population, especially among minorities (see, e.g., Morris and Hansan, 1995; chapter by Villa in this volume), with the possibility that future cohorts of the elderly will be less able to own their own homes. "Generation X" and the next cohort are not going to have the public policies, such as the GI Bill, incentives for broader pension coverage, and increases in the minimum wage, which enabled their "good times generation" grandparents to increase their rates of home ownership and retirement income and assets.

On the other hand, the financial status of the older population is still likely to improve over the next 25 years. Overall real median income is projected to increase from $15,523 in 1993 to $24,832 in 2018, while median housing and financial assets are projected to increase from $104,039 to $163,306. These increases may make it possible for the elderly to maintain or purchase better housing and services. Those aged 75 and older, however, will still have lower income and assets than the young-old, as will minority elders (Wiener, Illston, and Hanley, 1994).

This mixed picture of federal and state policies and the diversity among the future elderly seems to bear out the need for us to focus on elders aged 75 and older to ensure that the group of elders most in need of publicly funded housing and supportive housing policies will receive those benefits. Given today's political realities, however, it is not clear if we will develop and sustain the policies needed to ensure adequate and suitable housing for elders in the mid-twenty-first century.

References

American Association of Retired Persons (AARP). (1994). *A Profile of Older Americans*. Washington, DC: AARP.

Barriere, L. (1992). HUD's HECM demonstration program. Washington, DC: Federal National Mortgage Association.

Bass, S., Kutza, E. A., and Torres-Gil, F. (Eds.) (1990). *Diversity in Aging*. Glenview, IL: Scott, Foresman.

Cook, F. L., and Settersen, R. A. (1995). Expenditure patterns by age and income among mature adults: Does age matter? *The Gerontologist*, 35 (1), 10–23.

Day, C. (1990). *What Older Americans Think: Interest Groups and Aging Policy*. Princeton, NJ: Princeton University Press.

Dobkin, L. (1989). *The Board and Care System: A Regulatory Jungle*. Washington, DC: AARP.

Feder, J., Scanlon, W., and Howard, J. (1992). Supportive services in senior housing: Preliminary evidence on feasibility and impact. *Generations*, 16 (2), 61–62.

Golant, S. M. (1992). *Housing America's Elderly: Many Possibilities, Few Choices*. Newbury Park, CA: Sage Publications.

Golant, S. M., and LaGreca, A. J. (1994). Housing quality of U.S. elderly households: Does aging in place matter? *The Gerontologist*, 34 (6), 803–14.

Hawes, C., Wildfire, J. B., and Lux, L. J. (1993). *The Regulation of Board and Care Homes*. Washington, DC: AARP.

Heidenheimer, A. J., Heclo, H., and Adams, C. T. (1983). *Comparative Public Policy: The Politics of Social Change in Europe and America, Second Edition*. New York: St. Martin's.

Hoban, J., and Richardson, T. (1992). *The Local CHAS: A Preliminary Assessment of First Year Submissions*. Washington, DC: Department of Housing and Urban Development.

Home ownership. (1994). *State Legislatures*, 20 (12), 5.

Jacobs, B., and Weissert, W. (1984). Home equity financing of long-term care for the elderly. In P. Feinstein, M. Gornick, and J. Greenberg (Eds.), *Long-term Care Financing and Delivery Systems: Exploring Some Alternatives*. Washington, DC: U.S. Government Printing Office.

Lanspery, S. (1992). Supportive services in senior housing: New partnerships between housing sponsors and residents. *Generations*, 16 (2), 57–60.

Liebig, P. S. (1992). Federalism and aging policy in the 1980s: Implications for changing interest group roles in the 1990s. *Journal of Aging and Social Policy*, 4 (1/2), 17–33.

———. (1994) State units on aging and the implementation of the national affordable housing act: The results of a national survey. Los Angeles: National Eldercare Institute on Housing and Supportive Services.

———. (1995). State unit on aging efforts in housing for the elderly. *Journal of Housing for the Elderly*, 11 (2), 67–84.

Mackey, S., and Carter, K. (1994). *State Tax Policy and Senior Citizens*, 2d ed. Denver: National Conference of State Legislatures.

Mikleson, M., and Turner, M. (1990). *Housing Conditions of the Elderly in the 1980s*. Washington, DC: Urban Institute Press.

Mollica, R. L., Ladd, R. C., Dietsche, S., Wilson, K. B., and Ryther, S. (1992). *Building Assisted Living for the Elderly into Public Long-term Care Policy: A Technical Guide for the States*. Portland, ME: National Academy of State Health Policy.

Morris, R., and Hansan, J. E. (1995). A decade-long drift to public conservatism. (mimeo).

National Shared Housing Resource Center. (1989). *National Trends and State Initiatives in Shared Housing*. Philadelphia: National Shared Housing Resource Center.

Pynoos, J., and Liebig, P. S. (1995). Housing policy for frail elders: Trends and implications for long-term care. In J. Pynoos and P. S. Liebig (Eds.), *Housing Frail Elders: International Policies, Perspectives, and Prospects*. Baltimore: Johns Hopkins University Press.

Pynoos, J., and Redfoot, D. L. (1995). Housing frail elders in the United States. In J. Pynoos and P. S. Liebig (Eds.), *Housing Frail Elders: International Policies, Perspectives, and Prospects*. Baltimore: Johns Hopkins University Press.

Radner, D. B. (1993). Economic well-being of the old-old: Family unit income and household wealth. *Social Security Bulletin*, 56 (1), 3–19.

Redfoot, D. L., and Gaberlavage, G. (1991). Housing older Americans: Sustaining the dream. *Generations*, 15 (3), 35–38.

Regnier. V. (1994). *Assisted Living Housing for the Elderly: Design Innovations from the United States and Europe*. New York: Van Nostrand Reinhold.

Regnier, V., Hamilton, J., and Yatabe, S. (1991). *Best Practices in Assisted Living: Innovations in Design, Management and Financing*. Los Angeles: Long-Term Care National Resource Center at UCLA/USC.

Schwartz, D. C. (1984). Housing America's elderly: A state-level policy perspective. *Policy Studies Journal*, 13, 157–71.

Schwartz, D. C., Ferlauto, R. C., and Hoffman, D. N. (1988). *A New Housing Policy for America*. Philadelphia: Temple University Press.

Snell, R. (Ed.). (1993). *Financing State Government in the 1990s*. Denver: National Conference of State Legislatures.

Struyk, R. J., and Katsura, H. (1987). Aging at home: How the elderly adjust their housing without moving. *Journal of Housing for the Elderly*, 4, 1–192.

Struyk, R. J., Page, D. B., Newman, S., Carroll, M., Ueno, M., Cohen, B., and Wright, P. (1989). *Providing Supportive Services to the Frail Elderly in Federally Assisted Housing*. Washington, DC: Urban Institute Press.

Taeuber, C. M. (1992). Sixty-five plus in America. *Current Population Reports: Special Studies (Series P-23, no. 178.)* Washington, DC: U.S. Government Printing Office.

Torres-Gil, F. M. (1992). *The New Aging: Politics and Change in America*. Westport, CT: Auburn House.

Turner, M. A. (1989). *The State Role in U.S. Housing Policy*. Washington, DC: Urban Institute Press.

U.S. Congress, Senate Special Committee on Aging. (1991). *Aging America: Trends and Projections*. Washington, DC: U.S. Government Printing Office.

U.S. Department of Commerce and U.S. Department of Housing and Urban Development. (1993). *American Housing Survey for the United States in 1991*. Washington, DC: U.S. Government Printing Office.

Wallace, S., Williamson, J. B., Lung, R. G., and Powell, L. A. (1991). A lamb in wolf's clothing? The reality of senior power and social policy. In M. Minkler and C. L. Estes (Eds.), *Critical Perspectives on Aging*. Amityville, NY: Baywood.

Wiener, J. M., Illston, L. H., and Hanley, R. J. (1994). *Sharing the Burden: Strategies for Public and Private Long-term Care*. Washington, DC: Brookings Institution.

Chapter 5

Policy, Politics, Aging: Crossroads in the 1990s

FERNANDO M. TORRES-GIL

As the twenty-first century begins, issues confronting the aging of the U.S. population are at the top of the nation's domestic agenda. The assumptions and expectations of senior citizens and the reality of issues such as retirement, income security, employment, and health care will be profoundly affected by the political dynamics of the 1990s. In what way and to what extent changes will take place is still uncertain, but some images are becoming clear about the direction of policy and politics with regard to aging.

The programs, services, and benefits that have developed during the last 30 to 60 years will undergo profound scrutiny because of the political debates of this decade. The pending demographic wave—with the potential doubling of the older population—is creating a heightened level of public and political interest about how to prepare for, and respond to, the expectations of today's elderly and the concerns of tomorrow's older population.

This chapter looks at aging policy and politics in the latter 1990s from the prism of a Clinton administration's presidential appointee, and provides an historical and political framework by which to assess the direction aging policy might take and the issues and implications it raises.

Historical Trends

The last half century has witnessed the development of a series of laws, entitlements, and agencies that in turn led to an extraordinary system of programs, benefits, and services for older persons. The politics of the 1990s give important clues about the future of these public policies. The Clinton/Gore administration provides a vantage point for examining the crossroads facing aging policy.

President Clinton came into office at a time when aging programs and policies were well entrenched as an accepted part of American life. Medicare, Medicaid, the Older Americans Act (OAA), senior volunteer programs, Supplemental Security Income (SSI), and other programs had formed a safety net, albeit fragmented and complex, for older persons and their families. Yet the first term of this administration witnessed some profound questioning of, and changes in, those programs. To better understand the nature of those changes, it is useful to look back at the history of the policies during previous administrations.

The major social policies for the elderly—primarily the entitlement programs—were developed under Presidents Franklin Roosevelt, John F. Kennedy, and Lyndon Johnson. Social Security, Medicare, Medicaid, and the OAA came out of either the Great Depression and Roosevelt's New Deal or out of the New Frontier and the Great Society of the Kennedy and Johnson years. These entitlements not only reduced poverty and improved the quality of life for older persons, but they also became an accepted part of American social and economic life—so much that they enjoyed bipartisan support during Republican and Democratic administrations. The Carter administration, however, began to unravel that unquestioned support, not specifically for these major programs, but for the notion that the federal government should provide large-scale and centralized benefits and services. The criticism of government in general and of federal oversight and leadership in particular began to gain serious momentum during this time. The import of this changing view of government was not to be fully realized until twenty years later.

The Reagan and Bush years laid the foundation for aging policy and politics in the 1990s. This period saw intense efforts to balance the federal budget, to reduce federal spending, and to devolve federal responsibility to state and local governments. Values became an important part of social policy deliberations. Self-reliance, personal responsibility, volunteerism, and religion became cornerstones of the argument that individuals and families should be more responsible for taking care of themselves and others. In turn, the federal government would reduce its intervention—and, hence, funding—in both the public and private sectors. The extent to which the Reagan and Bush years succeeded in actually reducing the size of government and shifting responsibility to the state and local levels is arguable. What did succeed, however, were their attempts to change the nature of public discourse from support of large-scale entitlements to one that increasingly questioned the value of the federal safety net.

Aging policy was impacted by those debates during that period. For example, the 1981 White House Conference on Aging was notable for the controversies that arose over altering the Social Security system. The specter of generations competing for scarce resources gained credence in budgetary and congressional debates. Generational conflict became a watchword for those arguing that the elderly were receiving too many benefits at the expense of younger generations. Efforts to balance the federal budget (e.g., the Gramm-Rudman-Hollings bill), although unsuccessful, brought increased scrutiny on entitlement programs such as Medicare and Medicaid as well as other discretionary human service programs such as elderly housing and the OAA.

Despite misgivings about the size of the federal government and questions about the growth in senior citizen programs and benefits, there remained bipartisan consensus to refrain from radically altering the main entitlements—Social Security, Medicare, and Medicaid—and to provide continued funding to the potpourri of discretionary programs for elderly groups—subsidized housing and transportation, senior volunteer programs, OAA provisions, and SSI. The advent of the Clinton/Gore administration came at the point in aging policy when it appeared that there remained bipartisan support for the basic nature of those entitlements and discretionary programs and sufficient public and political support to retain them in their existing arrangements.

The Clinton/Gore Administration

When Bill Clinton was elected in November 1992, he received a majority of the senior citizen vote; thus the elderly formed a core constituency for his agenda. Indeed, during the campaign, he repeatedly stressed his support for preserving Social Security and Medicare. But his campaign speeches and appearances before senior citizen groups also carried a message of potential sacrifice and preparation for the future. He was not unwilling to tell audiences of older persons that they too would have to sacrifice for the good of the nation, and that long-established programs might need some changes in order to adjust to the priority of reducing the deficit and restoring economic security. The needs of younger generations and the imperative to invest in their education, training, and health care would be paramount in preparing for the future. In general, older persons on the campaign trail reacted well to this challenge, and the vote of 1992 showed that a majority of older voters were willing to accept the need to adjust to changes in aging policy, albeit with the security of knowing that the fundamental role and nature of public benefits for older persons would remain.

Focus of the First Two Years

The first two years of the Clinton/Gore administration were focused on addressing the core priorities of the campaign—the budget, health care, and welfare reform. During these two years, aging policy appeared to be of secondary importance. Yet the stage was being set for giving aging issues priority attention in the second half of the first term.

Health care reform by all measures dominated the agenda during the first two years. The extraordinary effort to dramatically alter the delivery and financing of health care consumed most of the administration's energy, although other priority issues such as deficit reduction and NAFTA also played a major role. After much effort the administration was able to pass a budget which, for the first time since President Harry Truman, reduced the deficit four years in a row. Welfare reform and the promise to "end welfare as we know it" saw the introduction of the "Personal Responsibility Act of 1994," an effort to dramatically change the traditional nature of welfare assistance and to set the stage for intense congressional debates about the proper balance of personal responsibility by welfare recipients and the insurance of an adequate safety net for the truly disadvantaged.

Health care reform, however, took center stage. The First Lady and her Health Care Task Force attempted to reshape the health care delivery system and to ensure near-universal coverage for all Americans. The administration's bill ultimately failed in Congress, but the struggle gave impetus to the concepts of managed care, health insurance reform, control of health care inflation, linking public and private systems of health care insurance, and streamlining Medicare and Medicaid—elements that would be revisited in subsequent debates on health care.

For aging policy, this health care reform saw substantial progress in promoting long-term care. As part of that effort, the president introduced a long-term care proposal that would, for the first time, provide a system of grants enabling states to establish home- and community-based services for older persons and persons with disabilities. The convergence of aging and disability interests and the recognition by the Health Care Reform Task Force and the administration that long-term care henceforth could not be seen just as an old-age program but one that would equally serve the needs of all persons who were frail and disabled regardless of age, was a conceptual and political breakthrough in aging policy.

While the campaign priorities unfolded in the first two years, other developments related to aging were occurring that would set the stage for the second half of the first term. Recognizing the cross-cutting nature of aging and the need to elevate the importance of aging in the Department of Health and Human Services (DHHS), President Clinton and Secretary Donna Shalala elevated the role of the Commissioner on Aging to that of an Assistant Secretary. This organizational change had both symbolic and real advantages. For the first time, the federal advocate for the elderly would have direct access to the secretary, the White House, and Congress, no longer being buried within the mammoth bureaucracy of the DHHS. The Administration on Aging, the federal program charged with providing community-based services, would be on par with other important federal agencies—the Social Security Administration (SSA), the Health Care Financing Administration (HCFA), the Administration for Children and Families (ACF), and Public Health Services (PHS). In addition, the assistant secretary for aging was charged with implementing the 1995 White House Conference on Aging (WHCoA), a seminal event previously scheduled for 1991 but held off in the Bush administration.

During Clinton's first two years, the Assistant Secretary for Aging was involved in both health care reform, especially the formulation of the long-term care proposal, and welfare reform. The Administration on Aging (AoA) was able to play a prominent role in the department's agenda by establishing initiatives on older women, long-term care, nutrition and malnutrition, crime and violence against the elderly, and development of a blueprint for preparing Baby Boomers for their old age. The role of the aging network—state and area agencies on aging, providers and volunteers, tribal grantees—became an integral part of the department's long-term care strategy with a closer partnership between HCFA (the traditional source of funding through Medicare and Medicaid waivers) and AoA (the primary provider of community-based services).

Political Earthquake of 1994

The elections of November 1994 were characterized by many as a political earthquake, altering the political landscape between the legislative and executive branches. For the first time since the Eisenhower era, both houses of Congress were controlled by the Republican party. Nothing had prepared the Clinton administration for this eventuality. The plans and hopes of the administration and its earlier agenda were now in jeopardy. How and why this political upheaval occurred remains a matter of much speculation and debate, one perhaps best left to political scientists and pundits. What was clear, however, was that the new Republican Congress, especially freshman members, saw itself with a mandate to radically transform government and to reclaim the Reagan agenda. Their "Contract with America" promised the American public a balanced budget, a devolution of federal authority and programs to the states, an injection of social values into public policy, and a dismantlement of the social welfare state.

Aging policy in this new order was to be a central element on the agenda in ways unforeseen by both Republicans and Democrats. The Republican Congress, perhaps based on knowledge of the electoral power of older voters, made it clear that its contract would not touch the Social Security system. Their contract also included some specific features that appealed to middle- and upper-income older persons: providing a more generous allowance in the Social Security earnings limitation test and allowing for senior-only housing. But beyond these specific age-related elements of the contract, the main preoccupation was to eliminate the deficit and provide tax cuts, and herein aging policy took a new turn.

The 1995 White House Conference on Aging provided a unique and unheralded opportunity to shape the political and congressional debate on aging policy in this new political environment (see chapter by Blancato and Lindberg in this volume). Although aging-related issues were not high on the initial administration agenda because of the need to fulfill campaign commitments, the WHCoA provided the impetus for the administration to once again demonstrate its commitment to older Americans and to support the fundamental role of Medicare, Medicaid, and the OAA for older persons. For aging advocates, the WHCoA provided a unique opportunity to assess and develop an agenda in this altered political environment.

The delegates to the WHCoA were a bipartisan mixture of individuals, having been selected by governors, members of Congress, national organizations, and state and local conferences. Although the conference operated on a relatively small budget and had limited time to be organized, it was by most measures a successful event, free of the overt partisanship that characterized the 1981 WHCoA. The priority resolutions provided a clear picture of the delegates' concerns. The top five resolutions included support for Social Security, Medicare, and Medicaid, and the OAA. The clear demand to preserve and protect Social Security, Medicare, and Medicaid was not unexpected, but the elevation of the Older Americans Act as an equal priority to those entitlements was a surprise, illustrating the growing importance of this relatively small program in the daily lives of older persons and their families who depend on its community-based services.

Initial reaction by some Republican members of Congress was to label the 1995 WHCoA a "pep rally for the administration." But in fact the conference included delegates appointed by Republicans and Democrats. The overwhelming consensus by both Republican and Democratic delegates was that these programs were fundamental to a social safety net for older persons and their families. This unequivocal support showed the administration that these programs were worth fighting for during the increasingly contentious budget debates. The 1995 WHCoA gave the administration a renewed opportunity to solidify links with senior advocacy groups and organizations that had not been uniformly supportive of health care reform efforts of the previous two years. During that time, many senior groups were ambivalent and even alarmed that proposed savings in Medicare, Medicaid, and managed care might somehow jeopardize the level of their benefits. But in a new Republican Congress, these same groups now felt that the very existence of those benefits were in jeopardy.

Budget Balancing

The budget balancing focus of Congress during 1995 and 1996 was unprecedented in its scope and its conflicts. For the first time in thirty years, a consensus had developed by all sides that the deficit posed a serious drain on the economy, that it should be eliminated, and that the inability to balance the federal budget would be a serious burden to future generations. The disagreements centered on how and when the budget balancing would occur. The Republicans proposed to balance the budget in seven years through major reductions in the growth of Medicare and through dismantling Medicaid as an entitlement. Discretionary programs would take major reductions in funding as well. In addition, a major tax break would be provided to middle- and upper-income persons and businesses. The president, on the other hand, while supportive of a balanced budget, vowed to protect Medicare from huge cuts and to preserve Medicaid as an entitlement while providing investments in other priority areas such as education, the environment, and human services.

Preserving Medicare and Medicaid became rallying points for senior advocacy groups and the disabled, while other interest groups—doctors, nursing homes, hospitals, and insurance companies—sought to work out their own deals with Congress to ensure that, whatever happened, their interests would be protected. Medicare, Medicaid, and other senior concerns became a bellwether for an administration seeking a clear demarcation between itself and the Republican party. Each side, despite the unprecedented turmoil and partisanship (including two government shutdowns), would use Medicare and Medicaid as their litmus test for selling a plan for balancing the federal budget to the American public. In turn, both sides would look heavily to senior citizen groups and older voters to gauge their reelection prospects.

Older Americans Act and Aging Policy

While this momentous battle ran its course during the first term of the Clinton administration, other developments took place that gave clues to the future direction of aging policy. As part of the congressional and executive branch consensus to achieve a balanced budget, discretionary programs faced major reductions and even elimination in some cases. Subsidized housing and and transportation programs (Section 202, Section 8, and transportation for seniors and disabled), food stamp and elderly nutrition programs, SSI, senior volunteer programs, and Title V senior employment programs, all faced severe fiscal pressures.

The focus on reducing the budget at all costs did, however, lend itself to some unforeseen opportunities for the administration and to the delivery of services to older persons and individuals with disabilities. The silver linings revolved around the Older Americans Act and the role of the aging network in serving older persons and their families. While Medicare and Medicaid took center stage in the budget debates, and while the 1995 WHCoA served as a platform for senior advocacy, the OAA underwent a major reauthorization. This reauthorization, having occurred on a regular basis since its formation in 1965, provided a rare chance for bipartisan discussion about the trends affecting an aging society and aging policy.

By the mid-1990s, political and public consensus had developed that large Washington-based bureaucracies were not the answer to the needs of local communities and individuals who demanded greater input, accountability, and participation in the allocation of public funds. The centralized categorical programs (e.g., Medicaid and Aid to Families with Dependent Children [AFDC]) were increasingly seen as overregulated, top heavy, and inefficient. Preference centered on flexible, local- and state-directed, community-based approaches to human and health services. Block grants and the funneling of public funds with minimal federal oversight and accountability were one response to this emerging public demand. At the same time, many questioned the propriety of block grants and the unstructured, no-strings-attached disbursement to the states, fearing that this would aggravate the problems of disadvantaged populations, especially in a climate of an overall decline in public dollars.

The OAA and the principles it embodied became a model for the delivery of community and long-term care services. Its services relied on local and senior citizen input through area and state plans; provided the bulk of its dollars to state and local public and private agencies but with national standards and accountability; had the ability to leverage its dollars by drawing state and local funds and voluntary contributions; and were flexible and adaptable to changing local and state needs. This tried-and-true system, with programs such as senior centers, home-delivered and congregate meal programs, ombudsmen, legal assistance, transportation, and information and referral services literally in every community throughout America, proved resilient and popular among governors, locally elected officials, Congress, and grass roots groups.

Long-term care and the move toward home and community-based services in lieu of institutional and nursing home care proved to be a crucial role for the aging network and the services of the OAA. Increasingly, proposals to expand long-term care would rely on the OAA and its infrastructure of agencies and social services to serve not only older persons who were frail and disabled and wished to remain in their homes and communities, but also caregivers and their families and younger persons with disabilities. This organizational and social trend signified a policy agreement by Congress, government officials at the federal and state levels, the administration, and service providers, which, to the extent that additional dollars might be available for long-term care, it should utilize the aging network, focus on community-based and social services, move away from institutional care, and serve persons of all ages with disabilities. The reauthorization of the OAA would provide additional impetus to long term-care and to the role of the Administration on Aging and the aging network.

In addition, under the guise of reinventing government, a prime initiative of the Clinton administration, the reauthorization of the Older Americans Act began the process of consolidating aging services under one administrative rubric, the AoA. For many years, aging services had been scattered throughout various agencies, including the Departments of Transportation, Agriculture, Housing and Urban Development, Labor, and Health and Human Services. With the pressures to reduce funding and the administration's initiatives to streamline government, an opportunity arose to begin the process toward a single point of entry and "one-stop shopping" for older persons, individuals with disabilities, and their families who heretofore had to deal with a multitude of programs, benefits, eligibility criteria, and administrative requirements.

The reauthorization of the OAA provided the chance to begin that process by proposing to bring the Title V senior employment programs administered by the Department of Labor and Elderly Nutrition Programs (ENP) administered by the Department of Agriculture into AoA, as well as other programs within and outside the Department of Health and Human Services. Thus, the federal government would make it easier for states and local agencies to do what many were already implementing—consolidating aging and disability services under one system and thereby making it easier and more efficient to provide services to consumers.

Lessons and Implications

What can be gleaned from the overview of aging policy in the Clinton/Gore administration? What are the lessons and the implications for the future of aging policy? Clearly, during this period, a momentous and perhaps long-term change has occurred in the relationships between the federal government, states and local communities, and the American public; changes that will heavily impact aging policy over the next 20 to 30 years. Several implications arise from these changes:

1. Policies and programs serving older persons are at a crossroads in terms of how they have served the elderly in previous years and how they may serve the next generation of elders. We are perhaps at the midpoint of a decade-long window of opportunity to prepare for a doubling of the older population and the political and social changes necessary to serve their needs.

2. Government is caught between two opposing forces: the demands of many to maintain the current system of benefits, programs, and services as they have developed over the last 30 to 60 years and the equally compelling demands of those who feel dramatic change is necessary in these programs if we are to be able to afford them later. Part of this dilemma centers around a public consensus that the deficit is bad for the United States and thus needs to be eliminated and an equally strong disagreement about how to do this. Voters made clear in 1994 that they wanted a balanced budget and a well-managed government, but when the specifics of budget balancing were presented the public made it clear that it did not want entitlement programs and services to the elderly, the poor, and the middle class to be eliminated or drastically altered.

3. This shifting and divergent public opinion has created a mixed picture for aging policy. On the one hand, support continues for Social Security, Medicare, Medicaid, and the OAA. On the other hand, expectations are rising that individuals must do more for themselves so that they do not become a burden to government and taxpayers. Saving for retirement, practicing good health, targeting and means-testing to the truly needy, requiring middle- and upper-income persons to pay more for government benefits, and promoting self-reliance and responsibility in preparing for a long life, will be central values that will define the level of public support for aging policy.

4. A critical reassessment of the New Deal and the social welfare approach from the 1930s and 1960s is underway and moving in the direction of drastically reshaping what has stood for many years. The details and potential changes are still very much uncertain. But the serious consideration being given to proposals to raise eligibility ages, means-test, or privatize Social Security, eliminate Medicaid and AFDC as entitlements, and reduce the role of the federal government in its oversight and enforcement responsibility, probably signal that aging policy will be much different in the first decades of the twenty-first century.

5. The shifting public opinion and this reassessment will put greater pressure on those who purport to influence aging policy—gerontologists, senior advocates, aged-based organizations, and consumers of these services and benefits—to rethink and, where necessary, to consider alternate ways to serve a population that will live longer and be comprised of a greater number of older persons. In turn, aging policy will need to incorporate changing public attitudes about what it means to be old, especially with people living longer yet feeling younger and enjoying better health in later years.

6. The debates of the 1990s cannot discount, however, that there will be a greater number of persons who will be at risk and disadvantaged as they get older, whether due to employment, income, race, health, or other circumstances. A social safety net still will be needed, but the question will be how and in what way it should be provided.

7. The diversification of interest-group politics revealed itself during this period. New aged-based organizations have developed (e.g., the Senior Coalition and the New Millennium) to argue in support of dramatic changes in entitlement programs. The traditional advocates in the senior movement (e.g., American Association for Retired Persons) found themselves under greater scrutiny and pressure to account for how they engaged in lobbying and interest-group politics. Even among older persons themselves, different priorities became apparent among those who were financially secure and those who were at risk economically.

8. Through all this, the much-studied Baby Boomer cohort began to voice its concerns about how they might age and whether or not they could expect to have the same level of benefits and services as their parents in old age. With the older segments of the Baby Boom approaching their fifties, they were becoming more engaged during the 1990s in the political debates about aging policy. Their immediate concerns continued to revolve around their parents and grandparents, how to afford the costs of health and long-term care, and how to care for their aging relatives. But with their old age clearly in sight, they will become a much more pivotal political and electoral force in the reshaping of aging policy.

Conclusions

The dramatic developments in aging policy during the 1990s have yet to fully unfold. But clearly, the future direction of this nation and our government's responses to the aging of the population is at a crossroads. Whether the existing array of entitlements, programs, and services will continue into the twenty-first century is uncertain. How to address the inevitability of more persons living to old age, with many doing well and many others doing poorly, has yet to be resolved. But what took place during the 1990s, particularly during the first term of the Clinton/Gore administration, lends important clues to the future direction of aging policy. We can probably assume that fiscal pressures and the public demand to reduce the deficit and to get America's fiscal house in order will continue well into the next century. But we can also expect continued disagreement and turmoil as the public, particularly the Baby Boomers, find that they too will probably need the services their parents and grandparents took for granted. How to reconcile diminishing public resources with heightened public expectations will be a defining dilemma of aging policy as we move into the twenty-first century.

Chapter 6

The 1995 White House Conference on Aging: A Tradition Confronts a Revolution

ROBERT B. BLANCATO AND BRIAN W. LINDBERG

> An older America must soon face a new century. The 1995 White House Conference on Aging allows us to plan for this challenge by working together to develop policy recommendations for the 21st Century. We owe this to future generations.
>
> President Bill Clinton, 17 February 1994

In officially calling for the 1995 White House Conference on Aging (WHCoA), President Clinton charged the conference with preparing aging policies for the twenty-first century. Indeed, White House conferences on aging had served as catalysts for aging policy for thirty-five years. The conferences of 1961, 1971, and 1981 prompted the establishment of major aging programs such as Medicare, Medicaid, the Older Americans Act, the National Institute on Aging, Supplemental Security Income, and Social Security Act amendments. The fourth White House Conference on Aging, held 2–5 May 1995, differed from its predecessors in a fundamental way. Instead of promoting new initiatives, it reaffirmed broad-based grassroots support for these programs. Why did the White House Conference on Aging precedent shift at the fourth conference?

The 1995 conference was conducted in a period of political turbulence known as the Republican Revolution. After the elections of 1994, the Republican party held a majority of seats in both the U.S. House of Representatives and the U.S. Senate for the first

89

time in forty years. The agenda of the Republican majority included promises of widespread reform in federal programs and a pledge to reduce the size and scope of government involvement in the lives of Americans. The 1995 conference was also the first ever under a Democratic president.

This political change influenced the products of the conference, as well as the process. It resulted in a pragmatic conference that emphasized the importance of existing programs, especially those that constitute the social safety net for the needy of all ages. This contrasted with earlier White House conferences on aging that were noted both for the number and scope of recommendations they produced. The first three WHCoA produced more than 2,300 recommendations while the 1995 conference produced 50 resolutions (synthesized down to 45 at the time of the final report).

The process of organizing and conducting the 1995 conference was also affected by the political situation. President Clinton mandated that the conference be intergenerational in nature and involve grassroots input. Not only was this a fitting charge for the conference that would set aging policy for the twenty-first century, but it was politically astute. An intergenerational approach to the conference would lessen criticism that a national conference on aging was too self-serving and one dimensional. To withstand potential criticism from conservatives and from the promoters of the Contract with America, the conference had to reflect the views of citizens across the country, not merely the scholars, politicians, and pundits of the field of aging and aging policy.

Therefore, the 1995 WHCoA involved grassroots activities as never before. The commitment to ensuring that it was a participatory process required that local, state, regional, and miniconferences be held before the main conference and afterward. In total, the 1995 WHCoA consisted of more than 1,000 grassroots events (800 pre- and 235 postconference forums) in all 50 states involving an estimated 150,000 persons.

The conference agenda, the adopted resolutions, and the implementation strategies around the resolutions were all developed in full consultation with the grassroots activities. While it is true that the focal point of the process was the three-day national conference that involved 2,217 delegates, 280 observers (including 37 international observers), more than 400 volunteers, and over 250 credentialed press, the work done by the many thousands of advocates, academics, consumers, business leaders, family caregivers, veterans, and volunteers before and after the conference was the heart and soul of the 1995 White House Conference on Aging. As a result, the 1995 WHCoA was a two-year long nationwide exchange of views on aging policy for today and tomorrow.

The political environment continued to influence the work of the WHCoA, and vice versa, well after the conference adjourned in May 1995. Medicare, Medicaid, and the Older Americans Act dominated the resolutions adopted at the conference and became the dominant issues in Congress throughout 1995.

Perhaps the best illustration of the impact of the WHCoA was revealed during the legislative action around the Budget Reconciliation bill that contained major reforms of Medicare and Medicaid. The bipartisan WHCoA delegates had voted, among other things, to oppose arbitrary cuts in Medicare and Medicaid and specifically to oppose using savings to finance a tax cut. Furthermore, they opposed ending the entitlement for services under Medicaid for children, the disabled, and the elderly. Immediately after the conference, the Budget Reconciliation bill was introduced and later passed by both the House and the Senate. It contained proposals for $270 billion in savings in Medicare and $154 billion in Medicaid in the context of a seven-year balanced budget. The proposal also called for a tax cut estimated to cost approximately $245 billion over seven years. Armed with the specifics of the budget, WHCoA delegates and others affiliated with the conference organized grassroots forums following the three-day conference to register their views on the budget and the impact the proposals would have in their communities. The net result was a strong call for President Clinton to veto the legislation, which he did. WHCoA delegate actions slowed the momentum on major changes proposed for both Medicare and Medicaid.

There are a number of other policy areas where 1995 WHCoA resolutions and grassroots advocacy have had an impact in congressional debates, including the Older Americans Act, the minimum wage, and the outside earnings limitation under Social Security. This, too, made the 1995 WHCoA distinct in that one did not have to wait two, three, or four years before seeing results.

The most important elements of the 1995 White House Conference on Aging may well be found in two of the messages it conveyed. The first is that while government is neither responsible for everything bad or for everything good, it maintains a fundamental responsibility to help those of all ages in need. The second and bolder message is found in the conference's effort to redefine aging—away from a focus merely on one generation to a focus on aging as a lifelong process affecting all generations. This redefinition must also be reflected in aging policy, so that decisions relative to Social Security, Medicare, Medicaid, and other programs are seen in the context of how they benefit the current individuals served by the programs, as well as the generations to come. These concepts may prove to be the most enduring legacy of the 1995 WHCoA.

Historical Overview

The White House Conference on Aging is the first White House conference of any type to be repeated more than twice. The 1995 WHCoA is the fourth of a series of such conferences. All four White House conferences on aging were authorized and appropriated funding by legislation passed by Congress and signed into law by the president. The traditional authorizing legislative vehicle is the Older Americans Act.

A forerunner of the WHCoA was actually held 11 years before the first conference, in 1950 by President Harry Truman. His National Conference on Aging suggested that the issues of the elderly in the United States would grow in importance in the years ahead. A major topic on the agenda of the 1950 National Conference on Aging was President Truman's proposal for universal health care coverage. More than 40 years later, planning for another WHCoA began with its focus on universal health care coverage, as proposed by President Bill Clinton.

The first WHCoA was held in January of 1961 in the last days of the Eisenhower administration. By the time the conference was held, John F. Kennedy had already been elected president, although not yet inaugurated, and his ideas were becoming well-known to the American public. They were reflected in the major recommendations that emerged from the conference, and in the ensuing years these recommendations became the programs now known as Medicare, Medicaid, and the Older Americans Act.

The second White House Conference on Aging, held in 1971 by President Richard M. Nixon, was the largest of the four with more than four thousand participants. Out of this conference came a number of critically important recommendations that paved the way for future legislation for seniors during that decade, such as the Older Americans Act nutrition program, annual cost-of-living adjustments for Social Security recipients, the Supplemental Security Income program, and the National Institute on Aging.

The third White House Conference on Aging was held in 1981, during the first year of the Reagan administration. The conference was actually called by President Jimmy Carter and the first two years of planning were conducted under his term in office, but the actual conference was held during Reagan's administration. It was a conference that featured its share of controversies, due primarily to the administration's injection of partisan politics into the process. One example is the last minute effort by the Reagan administration to add delegates that they had handpicked in order to "balance out" key state delegations and to avert having the conference repudiate administration policies. In all, the 1981 WHCoA produced a total of 663 recommendations. The most noteworthy of them provided the basis for the comprehensive Social Security reform bill of 1983. Other recommendations led to expanded home care coverage under both Medicare and the Older Americans Act.

The fourth WHCoA is the focus of this chapter and was called by President Bill Clinton on 17 February 1994. It was to have been held in 1991 under the terms of its authorization legislation, but the Bush administration failed to formally call the conference so it was not held (although more than $1 million was spent on planning).

The 1995 WHCoA Mandate

Congress mandated that the work of the conference be governed by a bipartisan twenty-five-member Policy Committee. President Clinton appointed Sen. David Pryor (D-AK) as chair. Senator Pryor was a close friend of the president, and at the time of his appointment he was serving as chairman of the Senate Special Committee on Aging. The Policy Committee met five times to approve the planning and agenda of the conference.

The authorizing legislation, the Older Americans Act amendments of 1992 and 1993 (P.L. 102–375 and P.L. 103–171), identified six primary purposes for the conference:

- To increase the public awareness of the interdependence of generations and the essential contributions of older individuals to society for the well-being of all generations;

- To identify the problems facing older individuals and the commonalties of the problems with problems of younger generations;

- To examine the well-being of older individuals, including the impact that wellness of older individuals has on our aging society;

- To develop such specific and comprehensive recommendations for executive and legislative action as may be appropriate for maintaining and improving the well-being of the aging;

- To develop recommendations for the coordination of federal policy with state and local needs and the implementation of such recommendations; and

- To review the status and multigenerational value of recommendations adopted at previous White House Conferences on Aging.

Preconference Grassroots Events

Of paramount importance to the 1995 WHCoA planning committees and staff was the involvement of as many individuals and organizations as possible—the grassroots community. In order to promote local, statewide, and national events, the WHCoA staff provided technical assistance to event planners, provided limited funding, highlighted upcoming events in its WHCoA newsletter, and attended events when possible. The WHCoA executive director, Bob Blancato, served as keynote speaker at many of the events.

More than 800 preconference events were held across the country, including all fifty states, Puerto Rico, the U.S. Virgin Islands, American Samoa, and Guam. More than 125,000 individuals participated in these preconferences. The events had to meet the following criteria in order to be recognized as a WHCoA event: focus on one or more of the federal policy issues affecting the elderly or near elderly, guarantee the participation of persons aged 55 and over, and present a written report summarizing the major issues discussed and the proposed recommendations within 45 days of the event.

The WHCoA office received more than 500 reports, with more than 10,000 recommendations, from the preconference events. The grassroots nature of these preconference events motivated the aging network to become involved in the development of the agenda. The process also produced new players in the aging world and involved both Republicans and Democrats. As the aging and nonaging organizations started to play more active roles and used their resources and numbers to conduct preconference activities, the WHCoA staff had to carefully weigh the networks' wishes against the voices of the "real people" who were attending events by the thousands across the country. Grandparents' concerns are an example of a set of issues that rose to the surface at the grassroots level and then were supported by the conference.

Preconference Grassroots Events List

Local Conferences (429 events) increased individual and group involvement at the community level.

State Conferences (59 events) encouraged states and territories to contribute input.

Regional Conferences (33 events) promoted regional collaboration among states on common issues and concerns of the elderly specific to their part of the country.

Miniconferences (260 events) addressed in greater detail specific issues and/or constituencies, for instance, older women's health.

National Preconferences (6 events) analyzed in detail and developed substantive recommendations for the conference agenda items.

Focus Groups (20 events) invited individuals of various backgrounds, ethnicities, educational, and income levels to discuss aging issues in small group, guided sessions.

All of the recommendations from these events were subsequently categorized according to the issues and subissues of the final agenda and were used later during resolution development.

Agenda Development

The first major role of the grassroots events, in addition to spreading the word about the conference, was to help formulate its proposed agenda. The development of the agenda for the 1995 WHCoA was carried out with the same attention to the voices of the grassroots as all other aspects of the conference. The WHCoA staff developed a comprehensive grassroots outreach program designed to identify key issues.

The first WHCoA preconference events are a good example of the commitment to grassroots and intergenerational involvement. The late Paul Kerschner, Ph.D., executive director of The Gerontological Society of America, organized forums in four cities in the spring of 1994. These events included panels of researchers, educators, and practitioners in the fields of aging and health care; focus groups of older individuals as a reality check on the agenda development; and a survey of all participants and attendees of the forums and focus groups to elicit feedback on support for a conference theme, specific agenda items, and viewpoints on various aging issue perspectives.

The initial discussions for the agenda of what turned out to be the 1995 WHCoA (instead of a 1991 WHCoA) began with meetings of a Senate Special Committee on Aging/House Select Committee on Aging task force established in May 1986. This task force consisted primarily of members of the Leadership Council of Aging Organizations (LCAO). They did not reach consensus on a theme, scope, or format for the conference, but unanimously supported having a WHCoA. There was some discussion on whether a conference could serve as a change agent and how this would affect the aging network. Interestingly, three key issues that the task force raised were (1) a need for more grassroots participation in the development of the agenda, (2) more focus on postconference activities, and (3) no prerequisite that conference planners restrict the scope of the conference because of fiscal restraints that might make policy recommendations impossible (e.g., the cost of long-term care). As it turned out nine years later, the conference did focus on grassroots and postconference activities, but the scope of the conference's recommendations (if not the agenda) was significantly constrained by tight fiscal restraints and the new political environment.

The WHCoA Policy Committee used a wide variety of sources to draft a proposed agenda, gathering input from local and statewide preconferences, past White House conferences on aging, and national aging organizations and individuals. Furthermore, once the recommendations and input from these sources were compiled and analyzed, they were published in the *Federal Register* on 12 October 1994, as the proposed agenda. The public was invited to comment on 19 major issues, 123 subissues, and 4 proposed conference themes by 1 December 1994.

The WHCoA Policy Committee reviewed more than 900 comments from individuals and organizations regarding the conference agenda. The policy committee developed a final agenda that consisted of 4 major issues and 22 subissues. The committee also selected the conference theme, "America Now and Into the 21st Century: Generations Aging Together with Independence, Opportunity, and Dignity." The final agenda, procedures for adopting resolutions at the conference, and the new theme were published in the *Federal Register* on 2 February 1995.

Following the agenda development, the WHCoA planning committees then focused their attention on resolution development and selecting the delegates who would come to Washington to participate in the conference.

Table 6.1
Final Agenda for the 1995 WHCoA

Major Issues and Their Subissues

I. *Assuring comprehensive health care, including long-term care*
   a. Promotion and prevention
   b. Access to quality care
   c. Continuum of care integrating community and social services
   d. Medicare/Medicaid/Older Americans Act
   e. Research and education

II. *Promoting economic security*
   a. Employment
   b. Social Security
   c. Other retirement income and resources, including pension reform
   d. Poverty and hunger
   e. Tax policy
   f. Discrimination

III. *Maximizing housing and support service options*
   a. Range of options/availability
   b. Affordability/financing/tax policies
   c. Linking support services to housing
   d. Consumer choice/decision-making/promoting independence

IV. *Maximizing options for a quality life*
   a. Resources for elders (community and social services/activities)
   b. Crime, personal safety, and elder abuse
   c. Spiritual well-being, ethics, values, and roles
   d. Image and roles of older people
   e. Elders as resources and opportunities for volunteering
   f. Isolation and loneliness
   g. Legal issues

Resolution Development

The planners of the WHCoA wanted the proceedings to be fully participatory but the final products to be prioritized. In order to keep the results of the 1995 WHCoA in a usable form, it was determined that delegates would chose a limited number of resolutions instead of recommendations. As noted earlier, the first three WHCoA had put forth 2,300 recommendations.

The 4 major issues and 22 subissues of the final agenda were used as the organizing framework for resolution development. A Steering Committee was formed for each of the 4 major issue areas. Members for the four committees were drawn from the Policy and Advisory committees. The Steering committees generated 60 resolutions for the 1995 national WHCoA using the 10,000 recommendations and 500 reports submitted as a result of the pre-conference grassroots events. The 60 resolutions were sent to conference delegates in April 1995, although the Steering committees continued to review and add resolutions until the start of the national conference in May 1995. Resolutions were also introduced by delegates at the conference itself (see the following section).

In addition, a Resolutions Committee was formed consisting of select members of the Policy and Advisory committees and the chairs of the four Steering committees. The Resolutions Committee developed the rules for the national conference, helped craft resolutions, and reviewed the draft resolutions of the Steering committees. At the national conference, the Resolutions Committee certified delegate-introduced resolutions that were to be voted on by delegates.

A list of the draft resolutions was sent to each delegate prior to the May conference in order to prepare the delegates for their work at the conference Issue Resolution Development Sessions (IRDS) (see the following section). Delegates were also able to introduce resolutions on issues that they felt were not addressed by the IRDS. The delegate-introduced resolutions, with signatures of 10% of the conference delegates, had to be submitted to, and certified by, the Resolutions Committee prior to being added to the updated list of resolutions on the ballot.

Delegate Selection and Preparation

Delegates to the 1995 WHCoA were responsible for voting on the resolutions presented at the conference in May 1995. Delegates were charged with helping to guide the future of national and state aging policy by setting policy priorities. Because of the important nature of the delegates' role, one of the most important functions of the WHCoA Policy Committee was to develop a delegate selection process. At its first meeting, 27 July 1994, the WHCoA Policy Committee approved a delegate selection process reflecting both nonpartisan and participatory approaches. Much attention was focused on the method that would be used to select delegates because of certain controversies that arose in 1981 around delegate selection.

The number of delegates was determined by two factors: the available budget for the conference (since the 1995 WHCoA continued past policies and provided travel and expense reimbursement for delegates) and the political composition of Congress and governors following the November 1994 election.

The Policy Committee of the WHCoA at its 5 October 1994 meeting approved an allocation of 2,000 delegates to participate in the May 1995 conference. The initial breakdown was as follows:

Chosen By	Number
Governors (State and Territories)	901
Members of Congress	540
National Organizations	300
Administration (White House, WHCoA committees, and staff HHS Secretary Shalala)	259

Governors who had the largest allocation of delegates were mandated to follow the matrix that had been established at an earlier WHCoA (50% persons over aged 55; 50% women; and percentages of urban, rural, and minority elderly equal to their percentage in the state) to help ensure diversity. Each state, the District of Columbia, and Puerto Rico were allotted six delegates, with American Samoa, Guam, the Pacific Trust Territories, and the Virgin Islands allotted one delegate each. Additional delegates were allotted to those states and territories with higher percentages of persons age 55 and older, compared to the rest of the nation. Age 55 was selected over aged 60 or 65 to ensure full participation by older minorities who on the average have a shorter life span than nonminorities. Members of Congress had total discretion in the naming of their delegates. They did not have to follow any age or population guidelines although they were encouraged to choose an older constituent whenever possible.

Delegates from national organizations were some of the more critical delegates chosen because there was an effort to achieve a greater variety and representation than ever before at a White House Conference on Aging. As a result, some of the 300 organization-based delegates included delegates from veterans organizations, youth groups, business and industry associations, volunteers, and those selected because they were caregivers. In addition, certain delegates were selected because they had conducted important miniconferences on specific topics that became part of the final WHCoA agenda.

In January 1995, the Policy Committee voted to amend its initial delegate allocation by allowing an additional 259 delegates to be selected. This was to allow the 97 newly elected members of the 104th Congress an opportunity to select one delegate each. The balance of the new delegates was given to the governors, allowing them 3 additional appointments thus ensuring that the 18 newly elected governors would be able to send delegates.

The reason for adding delegates to the 1995 conference—fairness—stands in stark contrast to the addition of delegates done just before the 1981 White House Conference on Aging. In that instance, delegates were added and selected to achieve a partisan purpose, namely, to ensure a greater Republican balance in key state delegations. The 1995 decision was bipartisan in its motives in that the overwhelming majority of those who were able to name delegates were newly elected Republican members of Congress and governors. Some have argued, however, that this decision made good political sense for the Clinton administration because it reduced the likelihood that the newly elected Republicans would oppose or criticize the WHCoA events or the administration's handling of the conference since they were now participating through their own delegates. Out of a possible 2,259 delegates that could have been selected, the 1995 WHCoA convened with a total of 2,217 delegates.

Because of the significance of the role they were to play at the conference, it was imperative that the WHCoA delegates be prepared properly and be aware of the issues and choices they would be expected to confront at the conference. To that end, the 1995 WHCoA delegates received a total of seven packets from the WHCoA office, five prior to the conference, and two follow-up mailings. The mailings contained information relating to administration (travel/hotel), conference procedures (rules, logistics, and voting), resolutions and IRDS selection forms, and background materials on the issues to be addressed at the conference. The background materials consisted of white papers written by experts in the field addressing each of the 4 major issues, 22 subissues, and crosscutting concerns, as well as demographic information.

As noted earlier, the 1995 WHCoA planners wanted to ensure that the delegates were informed in advance of some of the issues and choices they would be expected to confront at the conference. As a result, 60 draft resolutions were sent out in advance to all delegates. Out of this group of 60 resolutions, delegates were to select 40 that would be part of the group of final resolutions adopted at the May 1995 WHCoA.

The final mailing before the conference was a letter from President Clinton thanking the delegates for their commitment to the success of the 1995 WHCoA conference and to the future of aging policy.

The Conference

Ignoring and Exploiting the WHCoA

A valid case could be made that both the new Republican Congress and the Clinton administration largely overlooked the 1995 WHCoA in its developmental stage. Other than President Clinton calling the conference and nominating individuals to serve on the Policy and Advisory committees, there was little direct involvement by the White House in the planning of the conference. This may have been, in part, to avoid the criticism directed against the Reagan administration for their efforts to politicize the 1981 conference. Other than issues related to increasing the number of delegates to reflect the new political landscape, the direction and agenda of the 1995 WHCoA came as planned from the thousands of grassroots-based organizations and individuals.

This passivity of the legislators and the administration ended just before the WHCoA formally convened on 2 May 1995. The week before the conference, the Republican leadership announced that it would not release the specifics of their new balanced budget proposal until after the delegates to the WHCoA had departed Washington, D.C. Added to this climate was an interview given by House Speaker Newt Gingrich on the weekend before the WHCoA where he predicted that major Medicare reform legislation would pass Congress by September 1995. The speaker called on the president to use the WHCoA to help achieve a consensus on Medicare.

In a move to ensure more extensive media coverage, President Clinton addressed the opening plenary session of the WHCoA on Wednesday, 3 May 1995. The White House chose to have Vice President Gore introduce the president and to address the delegates the next night (the vice president was introduced by his wife, Tipper). In addition, First Lady Hillary Rodham Clinton conducted a plenary session on breast cancer prevention at the WHCoA. Two cabinet secretaries (Secretary Donna Shalala, Department of Health and Human Services; and Secretary Jesse Brown, Veterans Administration), as well as several high profile subcabinet members (including Jane Alexander from the National Endowment for the Arts), also addressed the three-day conference.

As the conference approached, there was also a notable increase in the intensity of activity on the part of senior advocacy groups. The rumors about proposed changes in Medicare, Medicaid, and the Older Americans Act were rapidly becoming formal legislative proposals and with that, concerns among senior advocacy groups mounted. In his address to the delegates, President Clinton seemed to recognize these concerns when he rejected arbitrary cuts in either Medicare or Medicaid that were done outside the context of genuine health care reform. He also announced Operation Restore Trust, an aggressive initiative designed to weed out fraud, waste, and abuse from the Medicare program, which was very popular with WHCoA delegates. The president's philosophy reflected a mood that spread throughout the conference: first, do not harm programs that are working successfully for older individuals; and, second, make only those changes that do not cost a great deal, that save money, or are cost-effective.

The media, especially the national media, were late to focus on the developing political drama at the WHCoA, due in large part to the tragedy of the Oklahoma City bombing just twelve days before the conference. The aforementioned comments by Speaker Gingrich served as a catalyst to get the media's attention. Regional and local media had already demonstrated their interest in the WHCoA since more than 800 preconference events had been held in the 50 states throughout the previous year. More than 290 members of the press were credentialed to cover the conference in its entirety. In addition, there was extensive coverage of President Clinton's speech as it was seen as a prelude to the rhetorical battles that would be fought between the White House and Congress over the budget and Medicare in the weeks and months to come.

Issue Resolution Development Sessions (IRDS)

The IRDS were the venues at the conference where delegates met to discuss, modify, delete, and approve resolutions. Each delegate could attend up to 3 of 22 IRDS presented at the conference; most IRDS were repeated three times during the course of the conference. The three-hour sessions followed a standard procedure for amending/approving the resolutions.

Each IRDS was staffed by two facilitators, two issue experts, two recorders/timekeepers, a room manager/monitor, and observers. A Steering Committee for each of the four major issues and two parliamentarians were available to each IRDS for technical support. This staff was responsible for the orderly conduct of business and for keeping the discussion focused on the appropriate resolution. The delegates could turn to the issue experts for guidance or clarification on points of information. This system enabled a great deal of discussion, prioritizing, and voting to be accomplished in a short period of time.

Once the conference was convened, all of the delegates were assigned to the Issue Resolution Development sessions (preferences sent in advance were honored to the maximum extent possible). These sessions proved to be the very heart of the conference and the very essence of the democracy that characterized the process. The selection of IRDS by delegates proved to be important to a number of advocacy groups since changes to the proposed resolutions had to be adopted by multiple IRDS to be able to be voted on by the full conference. As it turns out, those groups who deployed their delegates strategically within IRDS fared better with final resolutions. Some regretted that they had not developed strategies to ensure that their pet resolutions would be passed by each IRDS that considered it.

The policy and political priorities evidenced in the IRDS mirrored the priorities revealed through the preconference forums and also paralleled the growing concerns of delegates. These IRDS priorities were in essence to protect and defend existing major aging programs from reforms that would strip them of their scope and effectiveness.

The resolutions adopted at an IRDS were then sent to the parent Issue Resolution steering committee. The steering committee for each of the four major issue areas and their subissues analyzed the resolutions for duplication and germaneness and consolidated and reformatted the resolutions, as necessary. The resolutions were then forwarded to the full Resolutions Committee in preparation for the final voting on the last day of the conference. Many who participated in the IRDS process found it democratic and were gratified by the full participation of all.

Resolutions from the Floor

Delegates had an opportunity to introduce their own resolutions "from the floor." Each delegate-introduced resolution had to have the signatures of 10% of the delegates registered at the conference. The Resolutions Committee certified 39 delegate-introduced resolutions that were voted on, along with the other 59 resolutions, on Friday morning of the conference.

The products of these delegate-sponsored resolutions were also related to developments that took place just before and in the early phases of the conference. Again the future of Medicare and Medicaid and the Older Americans Act proved to be the fuel leading to the development of these floor resolutions. In addition, an inspiring opening day speech by the renowned aging advocate, the late Dr. Arthur Flemming, calling on the delegates to adopt a new intergenerational national community that honored commitments already made, served as a powerful motivation for the delegates.

The delegate-sponsored resolutions produced 39 choices for the ballot. In the end, a total of 10 received the requisite number of delegate votes to be part of the final 50 resolutions. These 10 delegate-sponsored resolutions included strong new resolutions reaffirming support for Medicare, Medicaid, long-term care, the Older Americans Act, more employment for seniors, and improved housing services. Those resolutions that failed to garner sufficient votes represent important statements unto themselves and are worthy of closer review in the development of future aging policies. They include topics such as expanded long term care coverage, more support for arts and elderly programs, and a call for the reinstatement of the House Select Committee on Aging.

The Voting Process

The last step in the WHCoA process, the voting on final resolutions, provided some of the genuine drama associated with the conference. It began with the internal processes that led to the preparation of the materials and ballots with which delegates would vote. The WHCoA staff faced impossible odds to reconcile all the changes to resolutions produced in the IRDS sessions and to continue to gather signatures on delegate-sponsored resolutions and have them prepared: printing and Xeroxing deadlines were scheduled close to the time when voting was to begin and added pressure was the fact that the entire conference had to conclude no later than noon on Friday, 5 May because another conference was scheduled to begin in the same hotel that day.

The WHCoA staff finished their work, but there were still minor snafus associated with the voting process including insufficient copies of the resolution books and ballots. Resolutions were posted early Friday morning, the final day of the conference and the day of the vote. Each delegate was required to wear his or her identification badge to gain admittance to the ballroom (the voting site) and was required to have a red voting card when turning in a ballot. If the delegate did not turn in a red voting card with the ballot, the ballot was not accepted. WHCoA volunteers were stationed around the ballroom to accept ballots. Only delegates, press, and staff were allowed in the ballroom during the vote. A total of 39 delegate-sponsored and 59 IRDS-produced resolutions were presented to the delegates for voting out of which came 10 delegate-sponsored and 40 IRDS resolutions. Results were announced to the delegates in the final plenary session that day.

Following the closing session a press conference was held where both Chairman Pryor and Secretary Shalala outlined the key issues and recommendations expressed by the delegates through the voting process. They characterized the conference as pragmatic and thoughtful and focused on the delegates' willingness to take into account current political and economic realities. Extensive media coverage occurred during the conference and at its conclusion that also suggested that this WHCoA was distinctive from previous conferences because it was a political, action-oriented event with more realistic and prioritized goals.

Postconference Activities

With the close of the White House Conference on Aging on 5 May 1995, an entirely new set of tasks, activities, and events awaited the WHCoA staff and the Policy and Advisory committees and national, state, and local organizations. The resolutions and recommendations of the conference had to be disseminated, a final report written and published, and resolution implementation strategies developed.

The WHCoA Advisory and Policy committees worked together to review the resolutions adopted by the conference delegates. Their task was to eliminate duplication in the content of the resolutions. In addition, due to concern expressed by advocates, the committees also reconsidered several of the delegate-supported resolutions that had received many votes but that had not been formally adopted. The 51 resolutions were pared down to 45, with the final 45 resolutions stronger and more focused as a result of the committees' efforts.

More than 230 grassroots events were held after the national White House Conference on Aging in May 1995. Their purpose was to recommend legislative and implementation strategies for the resolutions approved at the national conference. Delegates and members of the WHCoA Policy and Advisory committees were actively involved in all of the events, either organizing them, speaking at them, or providing technical assistance. The events ranged in size from seminars attended by fewer than 20 people to conferences with nearly 1,000 attendees. The recommendations resulting from the postconference grassroots events were used by the WHCoA Policy Committee in developing its final report.

Conference delegates received two follow-up mailings from the WHCoA office after the conference. The mailings contained the adopted resolutions, certificates, and administrative information.

Another postconference activity involved dealing with those who were not pleased with the results of the conference. In one instance, after the conference concluded, concern was raised by organizations representing veterans. Despite their unprecedented strong presence at the WHCoA, veterans were unable to muster sufficient support for any of their resolutions on the floor. However, in meetings called by the WHCoA executive director and under a decision approved by Chairman Pryor, a decision was made to allow two additional resolutions into the final group because of the significantly high number of delegates who voted for them. One of these was a delegate-sponsored resolution sponsored by veterans organizations entitled, Giving Older Veterans Choice in Health Care. It supports permitting the Department of Veterans Affairs to retain third-party reimbursement including Medicare.

Conclusion

Revolution is defined generally as a momentous change in any situation. In the political sense, it means a sudden political over-

Table 6.2
Final WHCoA Resolutions

1. Keeping Social Security sound, now and for the future
2. Reauthorizing and preserving the integrity of the Older Americans Act
3. Preserving the nature of Medicaid
4. Alzheimer's research
5. Ensuring the future of the Medicaid program
6. Ensuring the availability of a broad spectrum of services
7. Preserving advocacy functions under the Older Americans Act
8. Financing and providing long-term care and services
9. Expanding and enhancing opportunities for older volunteers
10. Assuming personal responsibility for the state of one's health
11. Strengthening the Federal role in building and sustaining a well-trained work force grounded in geriatric and gerontological education
12. Expanding, coordinating, and targeting necessary services
13. Reforming the health care system
14. Promoting innovative strategies to encourage new models of supportive housing particularly housing which facilitates long-term care services
15. Expanding the coverage of existing food programs
16. Meeting mental health needs
17. Maintaining personal choice and autonomy
18. Preventing crimes against older persons
19. Prevention/wellness throughout one's lifespan
20. Preventing elder abuse, exploitation, and neglect
21. Expanding training and employment opportunities for older workers
22. Designing housing to maximize independence
23. Providing services in a full range of locations that encompass institutional care, home care/foster care, and community-based services
24. Increasing Federal funding for research in the areas of the mechanism of aging, diseases of older people, long-term care systems and services, and special populations
25. Developing alternative options for funding long-term care
26. Providing oversight and ensuring greater public and private pension coverage, solvency, portability, enforcement, and vestment
27. Setting ground rules for guardianship
28. Support for caregivers
29. Enhancing community participation
30. Maximizing transportation choices
31. Ensuring the availability of appropriate care, services and treatment
32. Preserving and expanding Federal and State elderly housing programs
33. Encouraging policies that support and reward the development of suitable and safe communities
34. Providing health care coverage that addresses basic needs, prevention and chronic disease concerns
35. Strengthening and coordinating the delivery of legal assistance to older persons
36. Ensuring quality care, services, and treatment
37. Promoting positive images of aging by sensitizing society to the value of older adults
38. Expanding programs to assess and address malnutrition across generations
39. Addressing issues related to grandparents raising grandchildren
40. Targeting Social Security and Supplemental Security Income benefits for frail elderly women
41. Protecting the rights of older citizens and legal residents against discrimination
42. Encouraging development and ensuring implementation of advance directives, such as living wills
43. Advocating for children
44. Defending and advancing critical public policies
45. Giving older veterans choice in health care and permitting Department of Veterans Affairs to retain third party reimbursement, including Medicare

throw brought about from within the system. These definitions aptly describe the Republican Revolution of 1994.

With the Republican Revolution, the very role of government was under attack. Many Republicans during the 1994 congressional elections campaigned on plans to reduce federal spending and to curtail the government's involvement in American life. The approach taken by the Republicans in the Contract with America was to turn over more control of programs to the states, in many cases in the form of block grants. This was designed to save federal dollars and to provide greater control and flexibility to the states. Congress also sought to create a balanced budget by cutting funding for many programs and proposed various tax cuts in order to spur the economy.

The upheaval in the political status quo produced by the revolution led to changes, responses, and reactions throughout Washington, D.C. Decades of philosophical and programmatic "business as usual" made way for demands of reform. The planners of the 1995 White House Conference on Aging, from the White House to the Policy and Advisory committees to the executive director, heard the revolutionary rhetoric and understood that it was not merely the voices of a few who were espousing reform. In response, the conference planning process was altered to involve the nation's citizenry as never before. Throughout the development of the agenda, the selection of delegates, and the conduct of the conference itself, participation of the grassroots was of paramount importance.

More importantly, the participants in the 1995 WHCoA, the 2,217 delegates from both major parties, were energized by the political turbulence of the Republican Revolution. They responded to the budget-cutting philosophy of the Republican Congress by examining their own philosophies of government size and involvement. They seemed to use the challenges to their trusted programs as opportunities to analyze them and to assess their impact on their own lives and on society. The delegates took into account the limited resources of the government, the burden of the federal debt and budget deficits, and popular sentiments for reform. As a result, the 1995 WHCoA turned out to be a vote of confidence for the current system of programs, laws, and funding that makes up society's safety net for the elderly, the disabled, and the needy of all ages. Historically, the 1995 conference may appear to be a poor cousin to its more productive brethren, the previous three conferences, but in its focus to preserve programs, it was quite successful.

The WHCoA delegates, although well aware of the great gaps between needs and services, worked to pass resolutions that would save the integrity of the Medicare, Medicaid, and Older Americans Act programs. They supported changes in programs if those changes would save money, strengthen the program, or even provide more flexibility, but not if the changes would lead to the programs' demise. The president also took this approach when he focused on Operation Restore Trust, a new program under Medicare created to eliminate fraud and abuse in the system and to free up more funds for appropriate use. The administration also worked hard to educate the delegates that there would be serious threats to the Medicare and Medicaid programs in the months ahead.

Some lessons can be learned from the pragmatic approach taken by the delegates of the 1995 WHCoA. The delegates told us through their resolutions not to defund or end programs simply to fix a budget or to make a statement when persons of any age need those programs. They asserted the importance of evaluating programs on cost-effectiveness. Programs are not simply expenditures; they are investments. Cuts today may cost the government (and society) more in the long term. The Older Americans Act makes a good case for spending limited dollars to help individuals stay independent and living in the community instead of spending large sums on institutionalization. The nutrition program makes sense because diet and malnutrition are some of the main reasons why individuals need nursing home care. Keeping just a few individuals from unnecessary nursing home stays pays for a lot of home-delivered meals. Delegates stated strongly through several resolutions that community-based care programs must be protected and expanded when resources become available in the future. Furthermore, delegates declared that saving money through the use of managed care is acceptable only if consumer protections and quality are not destroyed in the process.

Aging research is another excellent example of expenditures that bring valuable returns on investment. Research helps to answer complicated questions about Alzheimer's disease, osteoporosis, incontinence, and thousands of other diseases and illnesses that lead to expensive treatments and poor quality of life. Delegates conveyed this and were not willing to give up hope or support for research on aging diseases and issues.

With this new political climate have come new members of Congress who are not prepared to make educated decisions about aging policy. There is a need and, from some, a demand for education. In the past, we have had enlightened leaders in Congress (Rep. Claude Pepper; and Senators John Heinz, David Pryor, and William Cohen) who understood the needs of those older Americans who wanted to work past the age of 70, those who were being forced out of hospitals sicker and quicker, and those who were living in board and care facilities that were regulated less than dog kennels. Today, we face the challenge of bringing our newly elected officials up to speed on the issues to which gerontologists and advocates are committed to regardless of the current year's budget woes.

We must also consider the basic political realities of the future. The aging population of the future will have many components and it will be ethnically diverse. There is a need to reach out to these communities if we as policymakers are going to be responsive to the needs of all the elderly. Women's issues will be at the forefront of aging policy because older women of the next century will have held many more leadership roles in our society and will be better equipped to advocate for themselves and for others. Delegates of the 1995 WHCoA acknowledged and reflected the changing makeup of the aging population.

White House Conferences on Aging in the past have led to legislative and attitudinal changes that have contributed to reducing the number of older individuals living in poverty, increased the number of older persons who have health care, improved the overall health of the elderly, and provided more access to long-term care services. Long-term care does remain the missing link in coverage for the elderly, and this was a major topic of concern during the conference. In fact, under different circumstances, the creation of a detailed resolution to deal with the issue of long-term care would probably have been the focal point of the conference.

Advocates will need to develop strategies to work within the constraints of the political and economic realities of the future to address long-term care and other critical issues for the elderly. This process needs to begin now and should be a natural extension of the 1995 WHCoA and its grassroots and intergenerational approach. It should also reflect the pragmatic and thoughtful work of the 1995 WHCoA delegates.

The 1995 White House Conference on Aging released its final report on 6 March 1996, and ceased operations on 31 March 1996.

Chapter 7

The Changing Political Activism Patterns of Older Americans: "Don't Throw the Dirt Over Us Yet"

SUSAN MACMANUS AND KATHRYN DUNN TENPAS

They stereotype seniors. They make it sound as if we sit and do nothing, like we are has-beens. I personally think we are a pretty well-informed group. . . . We may be over 65, but no one has thrown the dirt over us. They make it sound like once you get to 75 or 80, you don't have a thought in your head.

—Dorothy Romano, 68, Pinellas Park, FL AARP/VOTE
(Cutter, 1995)

As this quote from a senior rightly points out, stereotypes abound about the role of today's elderly in politics. Many of these emerged from research conducted a decade or more ago—when the expected life span was shorter, the roles of older women in politics and society were different, and there were fewer in-home options for political participation (Glenn, 1974; Pratt, 1976; Hudson and Strate, 1985). In this chapter, we examine the political behavior of the elderly by addressing the following questions: Are the elderly more engaged in, and informed about, politics than ever before? To what extent do they register, vote, participate in political party and interest group activities, contact elected officials (either directly or indirectly), and contribute money to influence the political process? How closely do they follow politics and what sources do they use? In short, our analysis shows that seniors are an even stronger force in American politics than they were several decades ago. To demonstrate these

111

points, we draw many parallels to the younger generation's political behavior. This comparison boldly illustrates why the elderly have a disproportionate impact on the political agenda. The key question for the twenty-first century will not be whether seniors will continue to be politically active, but rather whether their clout will weaken as the group becomes more diverse. (For an excellent overview of this expected trend, see U.S. Bureau of the Census 1992; McKenzie, 1993; Peterson and Somit, 1994.)

Registration and Voting

Older citizens register and vote at considerably higher rates than do our nation's younger cohorts (Table 7.1). Over three-fourths of the persons aged 65 and older are registered to vote, according to statistics gathered by the U.S. Bureau of the Census. Slightly lower percentages report that they actually vote.

Table 7.1 counters the once widely accepted disengagement thesis. This theory, first espoused by Cumming and Henry (1961) asserted that as individuals age, they begin to withdraw from various social activities, especially those requiring a significant level of physical and psychological involvement.[1] Recently, however, the proportion of the persons aged 75 and older who say they vote has risen considerably, thereby challenging the notion that older persons begin disengaging from politics in their mid-60s when they reach retirement age. "Indeed, where aging was once thought to automatically bring about a 'disengagement' from participatory roles, continuity of social participation and behavioral style across life stages is now recognized as the modal pattern of normal adult development and aging" (Steckenrider and Cutler, 1989, 66). While there is still some support for this thesis, especially when it pertains to the more demanding types of political activity (Jirovec and Erich, 1992), the age of disengagement is now closer to the mid-70s. It is likely to climb even higher as our society ages and as more mechanisms for nonphysically demanding political participation emerge (MacManus, 1996b).

Historically, women have participated less in politics than their male counterparts—a pattern usually attributed to socialization and educational differences and to higher incidences of physical infirmities among older women, especially widows (Peterson and Somit, 1992). Past research has also shown that older married women are socially and politically engaged longer than widows (Straits, 1990). Overall, however, the gender gap has closed considerably in recent

Table 7.1
National Registration and Turnout Rates (as Percent of Voting Age Population): 1972–1994, Presidential and Congressional (Midterm) Election Years

Registration Rates

Percentage Reporting They Registered

	Presidential Election Years						Congressional Election Years					
	1972 (%)	1976 (%)	1980 (%)	1984 (%)	1988 (%)	1992 (%)	1974 (%)	1978 (%)	1982 (%)	1986 (%)	1990 (%)	1994 (%)
Age												
18–20	58	47	45	47	45	48	36	35	35	35	35	37
21–24	59	55	53	54	51	55	45	45	48	47	43	45
25–34	68	62	62	63	58	61	54	56	57	56	52	51
35–44	74	70	71	71	69	69	66	67	68	68	66	63
45–64	79	76	76	77	76	75	73	74	76	75	71	71
65 and under	75	71	75	77	78	78	70	73	75	77	77	76

Sources: U.S. Bureau of the Census, Current Population Reports, *Voting and Registration in the Elections of November 1976, 1978, 1980, 1982, 1984, 1986, 1988, 1990, 1992, 1994.* (Washington, DC: U.S. Government Printing Office), Series P–20.

Voter Turnout Rates

Percentage Reporting They Voted

	Presidential Election Years						Congressional Election Years					
	1972	1976	1980	1984	1988	1992	1974	1978	1982	1986	1990	1994
Age												
18–20	48	38	36	37	33	38	20	20	20	19	18	16
21–24	50	46	43	44	38	46	26	26	28	24	22	22
25–34	59	55	55	55	48	53	37	38	40	35	34	32
35–44	66	63	64	64	61	64	49	50	52	49	48	46
45–64	70	69	69	70	68	70	56	59	62	59	75	56
65–74	68	66	69	72	73	74	56	60	65	65	64	64
75 and older	56	55	58	61	62	65	44	48	52	54	54	56

Sources: U.S. Bureau of the Census, Current Population Reports, *Voting and Registration in the Elections of November 1976, 1978, 1980, 1982, 1984, 1986, 1988, 1990, 1992, 1994.* (Washington, DC: U.S. Government Printing Office), Series P–20.

years as stereotypes about the proper role of women in politics and
society at-large have been reassessed. In recent elections, women
have even surpassed men in their turnout to vote.

The gap between older male/female registration and voting has
also narrowed. Between 1972 and 1993, the gap in registration rates
was nearly halved, dropping from 10.6% to 5.4% (Table 7.2). Older
voters (males and females) *consistently* vote. Seniors, especially those
who are active, tend to vote in all types of elections (national, state,
and local) and on all the races and issues on a particular ballot
(Miles, 1995). A survey taken in late October 1995 by the Times
Mirror Center for The People and The Press found that among persons aged 65 or older, 66.8% said they "always" voted and another
21.4% said they "nearly always" did. The comparable figures for voters
18 to 29 years of age were 21.5% and 29.8% respectively.[2] Other
studies have found that older voters are also more likely to vote in
all of the political races and on all the issues on a ballot. In other
words, they are less likely to engage in ballot roll-off or a voter's
tendency to ignore lower profile contests and referenda issues typically found at the end of the ballot (MacManus and Morehouse, 1995).

Not surprising, the greater propensity of older citizens to vote
in state and local elections gives them a much higher level of clout
relative to their proportional makeup of the registration pool than
exists in national elections. (In national elections, the turnout gap
between older and younger voters is narrower, although still significant.) Nowhere is the clout of elders in subnational elections more
obvious than in Florida. Overall, older voters make up nearly 40%

Table 7.2
Older Male and Female Registration Rate
Differences Shrinking

Year	Male (%)	Female (%)	Difference (Male-Female)
	% Registered Persons 65 Years and Older		
1968	81.7	71.1	10.6
1972	81.9	71.1	10.8
1976	76.6	67.8	8.8
1980	78.8	71.6	7.2
1984	80.2	74.7	5.5
1988	81.6	76.1	5.5
1992	81.1	75.7	5.4

Source: Jerry T. Jennings, *Voting and Registration in the Election of November 1992*
(Washington DC: Bureau of the Census, U.S. Department of Commerce, Current
Population Report P20–466, April 1993).

of that state's registrants. But on Election Day, they often make up an even greater proportion as was evident in a series of school tax referenda held in several counties across the state in the fall of 1995 (MacManus, 1996c). As shown in Table 7.3, disproportionately higher

Table 7.3
The Elderly's Greater Clout on Election Day, Florida County School Tax Referenda, 1995

County/Age Categories	% of All Registrants	& of All Referendum Voters
Failed		
Broward		
18–20	2.7	0.6
21–35	23.1	3.2
36–54	33.5	42.2
55–64	10.6	11.7
65 +	30.1	42.3
Hillsborough		
18–20	2.9	0.7
21–29	15.4	4.6
30–55	52.7	50.7
56–64	10.1	14.7
65 +	18.9	29.2
Leon		
18–20	3.6	1.1
21–29	26.4	8.6
30–55	46.2	58.5
56–64	11.5	12.1
65 +	12.2	19.8
Pasco		
18–29	11.4	3.2
30–49	28.0	23.3
50–64	18.7	21.1
65 +	41.9	52.4
Pinellas		
18–24	NA	1.2
24–55	NA	17.2
45–64	NA	32.6
65+	NA	48.9
missing	NA	.1

Notes: NA= not available. Supervisors of these counties do not report age break-downs. Data supplied by County Supervisors of Elections.

Source: Susan A. MacManus, "The Widening Gap Between Florida's Schools and Their Communities: Taxes and a Changing Age Profile" (paper presented at The Reubin O'D. Askew Institute Conference on Four Regions in Search of a State: Building Community at the State and Local Level in Florida. Gainesville: University of Florida, 9–11 November 1995).

numbers of seniors took the time to vote on these propositions in spite of the fact that younger and middle-aged persons (with children) had more to gain in terms of direct services. Older voters cited the current inefficiencies and ineffectiveness of the public school system as reasons for opposing the tax increase. More specifically, they thought that too much money was going to administrators and not enough to educators and the classroom. In addition, older voters, like persons of other ages, by and large think that taxes are high enough and are likely to oppose local tax increases of any kind (MacManus, 1996c).

Why do so many more older persons register to vote? There are several common answers to this question. First, a higher proportion of older persons than younger ages regard it as their civic duty to vote. Some attribute this sense of civic mindedness to their generation's prior education, especially the curriculum's emphasis on citizenship. Second, more believe that voting is an effective way to influence public policy. Since they are older, these voters are more likely to have had an opportunity to partake in politics and, more importantly, to have witnessed the impact of their participation. Third, the elderly are more likely to be strong political party identifiers, a factor found to prompt turnout. With age, one's identification with institutions (church, synagogue, and school) intensifies and the same is true for party affiliation. Fourth, they are typically more interested in politics at all levels and also more informed. The consequences of strong party identification and a familiarity with what parties and candidates stand for enhances their interest and knowledge in politics. Fifth, they are somewhat more likely to care which political party and candidate win an election. This phenomenon is a natural outgrowth of experience with politics as well as the fact that the elderly typically have more free time to learn about parties and candidates. (For an excellent overview of these points, see Texeira, 1992; Rosenstone and Hansen, 1993; and MacManus, 1996b.)

Peterson and Somit (1994) have conducted the most extensive modeling of turnout among the elderly. In *The Political Behavior of Older Americans*, based on data generated by the 1987 National Opinion Research Center (NORC) Survey, they test the influence of health status, stress, family size, marital status, church or synagogue involvement, and the standard socioeconomic variables on various forms of political participation. They conclude that "education, group involvement, race, sex, and age" are the best predictors of the elderly's political orientations and behaviors: more educated, involved, nonminority, male, and younger-old seniors are the most likely to participate (1994:79). In other words, the factors most commonly used to predict turnout among the population at-large are also the most effective at projecting turnout among its older component.

Participation in Political Party Activities

Involvement in "party politics" includes a broad array of activities: simply labeling oneself a party identifier; watching party-sponsored election activities such as party conventions, campaign ads, and candidate debates; giving time and/or money to a party or its candidates; or running for office under a party's label.

Identifying as a Party Member

Previous research tells us that as one ages, that person's party identification becomes stronger, along with their feelings toward institutions and family (Campbell, et al., 1960; Alwin and Krosnick, 1991; Jirovec and Erich, 1992). We also know that today's older citizens are still more likely to call themselves Democrats than Republicans, although the gap is narrowing for two primary reasons. First, there has been an increase in the number of older persons who label themselves independents, paralleling the trend across all age cohorts. Second, those who came of political age in the depression era are the most heavily Democratic. As members of that generation pass away, they are being replaced by voters who more weakly identify with the Democratic party or label themselves independents or Republicans (see Table 7.4). This is not surprising given relevant research on cohort analysis that suggests that political socialization rather than the aging process itself influences party identification. Rather than becoming more conservative with age, individuals have unique cohort experiences that serve as the primary influence on their party identification. Further demonstrating the trend of decreasing Democratic identification, data from October 1995 indicates that approximately 35% of the over 65 age group identified themselves as Democrats, 32% as Republicans, and 30% as independents. Another 3% said they had no party preference.[3]

Interestingly, the polls show that older men are more likely to identify as independents that older women: 32% compared to 24%.[4]

This pattern can be partially explained by the propensity of women to remain more loyal to their political party and to institutions in general (Peterson and Somit, 1994).

Many surveys have shown that older cohorts are more likely to see important differences between what the two parties stand for than younger voters. This should come as no surprise: "The passage of time offers people repeated opportunities to support verbally, and vote for, a party and its candidates, resulting in learning by means of psychological reinforcement" (Strate et al., 1989:453). Older voters are more prone to define party differences in economic terms, perhaps reflecting their years of experience with parties defined in such terms at election time (MacManus, 1996b).

Watching Party-Sponsored Activities

It is somewhat ironic that most Americans do not define themselves in highly partisan terms while at the same time, just about everything that happens during the election cycle involves the political parties to some degree.

PARTY PRIMARIES.   Primary elections are a political party's way of nominating candidates to carry the party's banner into the general election. Surveys have routinely found that nearly twice as many

Table 7.4
Party Identification in the 1990s: Persons 65 and Older

Party Self-label	November 1991 (%)	October 1992 (%)	August 1994 (%)	October 1995 (%)
Republican	33.1	28.4	28.4	31.8
Democrat	37.4	45.8	41.5	34.8
Independent	26.4	20.5	25.5	29.7
Other Party	0.3	3.7	0.1	0.1
No preference	–	–	3.5	2.8
Don't know/refused	2.9	1.4	0.9	0.8

Note: Respondents were asked: "In politics today, do you consider yourself a Republican, a Democrat, or what?"

Source: Telephone surveys of a nationally representative sample of persons 18 and older conducted by the Times Mirror Center for The People and The Press (now the Pew Center). Used by permission.

older as younger voters follow the primary contests rather attentively from beginning to end. The Times Mirror Center survey from October 1995, just a little over four months before the 1996 presidential primary season began, showed that 73.9% of Americans over aged 65 said they were "very likely" to vote in either the Republican or Democratic primary for president in their state compared to just 46.7% of the 18- to 29-year-olds.[5] The center's studies also showed that in both 1988 and 1992, over one-fifth of those 65 and older made up their minds about which presidential candidate to vote for during the nominating season—quite an early decision given that it is anywhere from 5 to 9 months before the general election.[6]

PARTY CONVENTIONS. In presidential politics, party conventions, held the summer before the November general election, capture the attention of missions of Americans. They are informative and entertaining, even though the party's nominee is usually a foregone conclusion by the time the convention rolls around. Most Americans follow the party conventions on television. They acknowledge that they are most interested in learning about the party platforms (mentioned by more than 70% of each age group). When asked about their interest in other convention activities such as the roll call of states, intraparty personality conflicts, and the nominee's acceptance speech, older voters are the most interested in hearing the nominee's acceptance speech. Between 6% and 12% of all older voters even say they decide whom to support for president at the end of the conventions, depending upon their competitiveness (MacManus, 1996b).

DEBATES. Candidate debates are even more popular events than party conventions. "The media's tendency to turn debates into boxing matches, proclaiming winners and losers as soon as the sparring ends, creates more interest than usual and enhances the media's influence" (MacManus, 1996b:83). Interestingly, these debates have a disparate impact on viewers. While they usually reinforce the opinions of older persons, debates tend to form or change those of younger voters (MacManus, 1996b). Across both age groups, debate formats that feature questioning by either voters or a single moderator are favored over those featuring inquiries by a panel of select journalists, usually from the national press corps.

CAMPAIGN ADS. Political advertisements are often sponsored by the national or state parties and, more frequently, by the candidates themselves. Advertisements are seen as an effective way to reach the potential voter without having to go through the press. They take many forms: brochures, newsletters, videos, home pages on the world wide web, billboards, yard signs, bumper stickers, newspaper ads, and radio and television commercials. A sizable portion of the electorate first learns about a candidate or a party stance from televised political advertisements. In 1988 and 1992, almost two-thirds of the electorate admitted that they first learned about a candidate or issue from these advertisements (68.2% of those 65 and older, 63.4% of those 18 to 29). And a postelection study in 1992 found that well over one-third of the voters credited ads with helping them decide for whom to vote (36.1% of the seniors and 43.1% of the 18–29-year-olds) (MacManus, 1996b).

POLITICAL PARTY GRASSROOTS ACTIVISTS. People who actually take part in party organization activities are much stronger party identifiers than those who do not participate. A large-scale comparative study of grassroots party activists in eleven southern states found that older party activists in both parties "are more likely to be involved in registration drives, the contacting of voters generally and new voters specifically, local candidate recruitment efforts, and county party organizational work and party business meetings" (Shaffer and Breaux, 1992:9) (see Table 7.5). Over 90% of the local county party Democratic activists who are 70 years and older say they are active in getting people to register, 87% contact voters, nearly three-fourths are active in campaigns and in party public relations work, and approximately two-thirds recruit party workers and candidates for local office.

RUNNING FOR OFFICE. Very few people ever run for political office (somewhere in the neighborhood of one out of a hundred). This form of political participation is the most demanding and perhaps the most physically and mentally draining. Additionally, it often takes a heavy toll on a person's time, family, finances, and privacy. Predictably, older Americans are less likely than younger adults to run for elective posts that take them away from home, especially from their grandchildren. Thus, when persons enter electoral politics late in life, they tend to run for a *local* government post, most often a city council seat in a small jurisdiction. Many have held leadership positions in community organizations before taking the plunge into elective office (MacManus, 1996b).

Other Forms of Political Activism

Political activism is not limited to registering, voting, and participating in party-related events. Americans often exert their

TABLE 7.5
Activities Performed in Current Party Position By Grassroots Party Activists

Activity	Democrats					Republicans				
	Under-40 (%)	40-49 (%)	50-59 (%)	60-69 (%)	70+ (%)	Under 40 (%)	40-49 (%)	50-59 (%)	60-69 (%)	70+ (%)
Contacting voters	82	80	84	87	87*	82	82	87	88	88*
Raising money	55	55	51	53	51	50	56	59	58	60*
Getting people to register to vote	79	79	84	89	91*	74	77	84	84	87*
Campaigning	79	74	73	73	72*	80	79	79	73	69*
Public relations	74	73	77	77	76	69	70	76	74	70*
Contacting new voters	72	68	76	80	81*	67	70	77	79	78*
Participate in Party meetings/business	81	79	83	85	87	80	80	85	86	87*
Recruiting and organizing workers	69	66	70	69	67	66	67	72	69	65*
County Party organizational work	67	66	72	72	71*	62	66	69	71	73*
Increasing political info for voters	75	74	76	76	78	76	80	79	79	80
Policy formulation	56	55	58	59	59	54	59	60	60	62*
Getting candidates for local office	60	60	63	68	65*	61	66	69	69	68*
Other nominating activities	46	41	46	47	40*	40	46	46	46	41*

Notes: *Indicates statistically significant relationship using chi square at 0.05 level. Data are from the eleven state Southern Grassroots Party Activists Project, a collaborative effort funded by the National Science Foundation and administered through the University of New Orleans.

Source: Stephen D. Shaffer and David Breaux. "Generational Differences among Southern Grassroots Party Workers" paper presented at the 1992 Annual Meeting of the American Political Science Association, Chicago, IL, 3–6 September 1992, p. 25. Reprinted with permission of the American Political Science Association and the authors. From Susan A. MacManus, *Young v. Old: Generational Combat in the 21st Century.* (Boulder, CO: Westview Press, 1996), p. 109.

influence on the political process by directly contacting public officials via letter, telephone, fax, or e-mail or at a public hearing or forum. Increasingly, they are also letting their policy preferences be known through more *indirect* routes. These are usually media based (e.g., letters to the editor, call-in talk shows, and instantaneous public opinion polls) (MacManus, 1996a). Often they join with others to exert pressure on the system, via petitions, protests, lawsuits, political action committees (PACs) and via other forms of collective activity (see Table 7.6).

Some forms of activism take more personal and physical effort than others. For many older Americans, difficulties with physical mobility make it far more preferable to engage in political activities that are home-based. For them, it is easier to pick up the telephone and call a city council member to protest a proposed policy than it is to attend a city council meeting. But it is interesting to note that if an older person attends a public forum, he or she is more likely to speak than a younger attendee. For example, a 1987 Times Mirror Center survey found that only 2.6% of the 18- to 29-year-olds acknowledged that they had spoken at a public hearing compared to 10.4% of those 60 and older.[7]

Times Mirror Center for The People and The Press polls have consistently shown that older persons are much more actively engaged as contactors and financial contributors than as protestors, meeting attendees/leaders, or petition circulators, suggesting that the level of physical exertion affects participation (Jennings and Markus, 1988; Miles, 1995). For example, Times Mirror Center surveys in 1992 and 1993 found that over half of those 65 and older reported that they had called or sent a letter to their Congress member, 27% contributed money to a candidate, and 17% contributed money to a PAC. In contrast, just 9% had boycotted a company and only 2% to 3% had taken part in a public demonstration.[8] A 1987 survey found that just 3% of those over 60 had initiated or participated in a lawsuit.[9]

There are other reasons besides physical mobility that explain why older citizens are active contactors and financiers. First, many have more experience dealing with government and thus know who and how to contact effectively. Second, they tend to be better informed about issues and about the timing of the political process. Third, a sizable number of retirees are in a sound enough financial position to be able to contribute to interest groups, political action committees, and candidates.

Table 7.6
Participation in Nonvoting Forms of Political Activity by Age Group

Political Activity	18–34 %	34–44 %	Age Group 45–54 %	55–64 %	65+ %
Direct Contacting					
Written a letter to any elected official	21.1	32.6	41.2	28.3	33.8
Called or sent a letter to your Congress member	23.5	42.9	48.0	50.1	53.9
Called or sent a letter to the White House	6.9	14.4	21.9	22.3	21.3
Indirect Contacting					
Written a letter to the editor of a newspaper	11.0	16.0	16.6	12.9	12.7
Called into a television station or cable company to complain about a program	11.3	9.9	9.5	14.4	7.6
Called in or sent a response to a question or issue put up for discussion by a newspaper or TV station	13.4	17.1	20.3	12.9	7.3
Tried to call into a talk show to discuss views on a public or political issue	7.9	14.7	5.9	7.8	7.6
Dialed an 800 or 900 number to register an opinion on some issue of public concern	14.2	20.6	13.8	15.3	10.1
Participated in a poll sent by a group one belongs to	22.3	33.5	38.9	31.2	19.8
Joining/Attending					
Joined an organization in support of a particular cause	19.9	24.9	27.1	20.1	15.2
Attended a city or town meeting in one's community	21.7	27.5	33.4	39.8	38.6
Attended a public hearing	27.7	34.4	43.9	40.6	35.6
Participated in a "town meeting" or public affairs discussion group	17.7	28.1	30.6	32.8	24.5
Contributing					
Contributed money to a PAC	8.9	17.5	16.3	18.0	17.0
Contributed money to a candidate running for public office	10.7	21.4	26.9	23.1	26.9

Note: Respondents were asked: "People express their opinions about politics and current events in a number of ways besides voting. I'm going to read a list of some of these ways. Please just tell me if you have or have not ever done each. Have you ever [X]?"

Source: Times Mirror Center for The People & The Press. Telephone survey of a nationally representative sample of 1,507 adults 18 years of age or older, conducted 18–24 May 1993. From Susan A. MacManus, Young v. Old: Generational Combat in the 21st Century. (Boulder, CO: Westview Press, 1996), p. 141.

Highly Attentive and Well-Informed

Older Americans are much more interested in politics and public affairs than younger citizens. An October 1995 Times Mirror Center survey presented its respondents with this question: "Some people seem to follow what's going on in government and public affairs most of the time, whether there's an election or not. Others aren't that interested. Would you say you follow what's going on in government and public affairs most of the time, some of the time, only now and then, or hardly at all?"[10] Over 59% of those over age 65 said they follow it "most of the time," compared to just 30% of the 18-to 29-year-olds.

In terms of news sources, older Americans rely on more, and different, types than the young. Times Mirror Center surveys have documented that a considerably higher proportion of seniors regularly rely on virtually all news sources more than their younger counterparts, except for television talk shows and personality magazines (the "lite" news sources) (see Table 7.7).

Among the elderly, 83% report that they regularly watch local television news, 75% read a daily newspaper, 75% listen to national network news, and 67% watch news magazine shows (see Table 7.7). They are traditionalists when it comes to news sources. In contrast, younger Americans are fond of daytime television talk shows that discuss current events they regard as "news."

Expanding the Political Involvement of the Elderly

Modern technology and legislative reforms will continue to expand the citizenry's opportunities for political involvement. Technological advancements accompanied by political reform will make it more convenient for the elderly to influence public policy—safely and comfortably from their own homes or congregate care facilities. One of the fastest growing ways to communicate with public officials (and with other seniors) is via the Internet. SeniorNet clubs are springing up everywhere putting a growing number of older Americans "on-line."

The mushrooming number of cable television channels has offered TV viewers a plethora of political news sources, C-SPAN and CNN being two of the more popular venues for watching national-level politics. Local public access channels bring city, county, and school board politics into the living room. Thus, it has become

Table 7.7
News Sources Regularly Relied Upon by Different Age Groups

			Age Group		
Regular News Sources	18–29 (%)	30–49 (%)	50–64 (%)	65+ (%)

	18–29 (%)	30–49 (%)	50–64 (%)	65+ (%)
ELECTRONIC MEDIA				
Television				
Local news about your viewing area	69.9	77.7	82.1	83.0
National network news on CBS, ABC, or NBC	45.6	55.5	72.8	75.1
Cable News Network (CNN)	31.6	33.3	38.5	40.8
Macneil/Lehrer News Hour	2.9	8.3	16.6	16.1
C-Span	10.1	10.5	13.7	12.4
Sunday morning news shows (such as *Meet The Press, Face The Nation,* or *This Week with David Brinkley*)	7.4	17.0	25.1	29.4
News magazine shows (such as *60 Minutes* or *20/20*)	36.1	52.0	59.4	66.9
Talk shows (such as *Oprah, Donahue,* or *Geraldo*)	34.6	21.5	22.6	18.0
The Rush Limbaugh Show	8.1	6.7	4.2	8.8
The Larry King Show	3.1	3.6	6.3	9.8
Radio				
Programs on National Public Radio such as *Morning Edition* or *All Things Considered*	13.0	14.1	18.2	15.3
Call in talk shows	12.4	17.1	22.8	15.0
PRINT MEDIA				
Newspapers				
Daily newspaper	56.5	65.6	69.9	75.4
Magazines				
News (such as *Time, US News and World Report,* or *Newsweek*)	18.8	25.2	24.1	26.4
Personality (such as *People* or *US*)	16.0	11.2	9.2	8.0

Note: Respondents were asked: "I'd like to know how often, if ever, you read certain types of publications, listen to the radio, or watch certain types of TV shows. For each that I read, tell me if you do it regularly, sometimes, hardly ever, or never. How often do you [X]?"

Source: Times Mirror Center for The People and The Press, Telephone survey of a nationally representative sample of 1,507 adults 18 years of age or older, conducted 18–24 May 1993. From Susan A. MacManus, *Young v. Old: Generational Combat in the 21st Century* (Boulder, CO: Westview Press, 1996), p. 54.

easier for older Americans to follow "live" politics at all levels of government on an almost daily basis.

The popularity of VCRs and videotapes have also made it easier for governments, elected officials, and candidates to reach out to the elderly, particularly those who are home-bound. To date, political candidates have used this medium most effectively. They send videotapes of their campaign messages to older voters in their districts (although the elderly are by no means always the only recipients) and/or to congregate care facilities. Using this technique, a candidate can connect with older or infirmed constituents who might not be able to attend a political rally or public forum.

As more Americans reside in retirement communities and congregate care facilities, we expect more candidates and elected officials to personally deliver their messages to such locations. In south Florida, condominiums are already a "must" stop for political candidates seeking the vital elderly vote. This trend will gradually extend to the nation at-large.

In addition to technologically driven ways of enhancing democracy, many states have sought to expand the electorate by passing new laws making it easier for older, infirmed Americans to register and vote. Postcard voter registration is now commonplace as is registration at drivers' license bureaus and social service agencies following the passage of the federal "Motor Voter" Act. Indeed, many states have already adopted laws permitting registration at driver's license bureaus before the federal law was passed.

A growing number of states have adopted "early voting" procedures whereby polls at key precincts (often community centers) are open several weeks prior to the actual election day. Many states also permit formal "proxy-voting" whereby citizens unable to travel to the polling place have a relative or friend help them complete an absentee ballot. On-site proxy voting is permitted in virtually every state for the sight and physically impaired.

Another trend is voting by mail that the State of Oregon has popularized and demonstrated can be both effective and efficient. We expect that it will not be too far into the future when: ". . . election laws catch up with technology and make it possible to register and vote electronically from a wide variety of locations (e.g., homes, hospitals, nursing homes, or other congregate care facilities)" (MacManus, 1996b:52). Finally, while it is still difficult for many older citizens to participate in certain physically demanding political activities (e.g., campaigning door-to-door, protesting, marching, attending legislative body meetings, and/or public forums), we expect many of these activities to become more electronically based as we move toward interactive communication modes.

Conclusion

Older Americans have always participated more in politics than their younger counterparts. But today's seniors are participating in a much wider array of activities and staying politically engaged much longer. Technological innovations (e.g., cable television, VCRs, facsimiles, and computers) have made it easier for older persons to communicate with public officials in the safety and security of their own homes. Furthermore, changes in state election laws permitting registration and voting via mail, proxy voting, and early voting have also expanded political participation. The pace at which our nation is aging will undoubtedly spark more technological advancements and legal reforms in the future.

America's seniors are also more experienced at contacting their elected officials and making their voices known than younger voters. They are more likely to follow politics closely; get their information from a wide variety of sources; donate money to candidates, interest groups, and political parties; vote in elections at all levels (not just in presidential contests); and vote for all the contests and issues on a ballot. Predictably, elected officials see older voters as a critical constituency base:

> Politicians can serve either the active or inactive. The active contribute directly to their goals: They pressure, they contribute, they vote. The inactive offer only potential, the possibility that they might someday rise up against rules who neglect them. Only the rare politician would pass up the blandishments of the active to champion the cause of those who never take part. (Rosenstone and Hansen, 1993:247)

The nation's younger cohorts are finally beginning to realize what elected officials have known for quite some time, namely that older constituents wield a disproportionate amount of political clout. The best evidence of their growing clout is demonstrated by the younger cohort's frequent complaint that politicians are only concerned with issues pertaining to the elderly (e.g., Social Security, Medicare, and Medicaid). The political strength of older constituents lies in their growing numbers, their greater propensity to participate at all levels, and in their willingness (and knowledge of how) to interject their preferences at each stage of the policy-making process. Contrary to popular stereotypes, our research reveals that seniors are fairly well-informed—and they are *unlikely* to sit and do nothing when the political winds begin to blow. However, there is little to suggest that all older Americans will set sail in the *same* direction.

Notes

1. For a discussion on the relevance of the disengagement theory, see Jennings and Markus (1988).

2. Telephone survey of a nationwide random sample of 2,000 adults 18 years of age or older, conducted during the period 25–30 October 1995. The margin of error was ± 2%. (Times Mirror Center for the People and The Press (14 November 1995). *Voter Anxiety Driving GOP: Energized Democrats Backing Clinton* (Washington, DC: Times Mirror Center for The People and The Press).

3. Telephone survey of a nationally representative sample of 2,000 voters 18 years of age or older conducted 25–30 October 1995.

4. Information obtained from a Times Mirror Center for The People and The Press telephone survey of a nationally representative sample of 1,819 adults 18 years of age and older, conducted March 1995.

5. Ibid. Respondents were asked: "If there is a primary in your state next year, how likely is it that you will vote in either the Republican or Democratic primary for president? Is it very likely, somewhat likely, not too likely, or not at all likely?"

6. Respondents were asked: "When did you make up your mind definitely to vote for [candidate you said you voted for]?" (open-ended question). The 1988 figure (22.7%) was for persons 60 years of age and older; the figure (21.8) was for persons aged 65 and older.

7. A face-to-face survey of a national representative sample of 4,244 adults aged 18 and older conducted in May–June 1989.

8. A telephone survey of a nationally representative sample of 3,517 adults 18 years of age or older, conducted 28 May–10 June 1992.

9. A face-to-face survey of a nationally representative sample of 4,244 adults 18 years of age or older, conducted 25 April–10 May 1987.

10. Telephone survey of a nationally representative sample of 2,000 voters 18 years of age or older conducted 25–30 October 1995.

References

Alwin, Duane F., and Krosnik, Jon A. (1991). Aging, cohorts, and the stability of sociopolitical orientations over the life span. *American Journal of Sociology*, 97, 169–95.

Campbell, Angus, Converse, Philip E., Miller, Warren E., and Stokes, Donald E. (1960). *The American Voter*. New York: Wiley.

Cumming, E., and Henry, W. E. (1961). *Growing Old: The Process of Disengagement*. New York: Basic.

Cutter, John A. (1995). Seniors don't scare so easily. *St. Petersburg Times*, 19 November, p. 1D.

Glenn, Norval D. (1974). Aging and conservatism. *Annals of the American Academy of Political and Social Science*, 415, 176–86.

Hudson, Robert B., and Strate, John. (1985). Aging and political systems. In Robert H. Binstock and E. Shanas (Eds.). *Handbook of Aging and the Social Sciences*. 2d ed., pp. 554–85. New York: Van Nostrand.

Jennings, M. Kent, and Markus, Gregory B. (1988). Political involvement in the later years: A longitudinal survey. *American Journal of Political Science*, 32 (May), 302–16.

Jirovec, Ronald L., and Erich, John. (1992). Dynamics of political participation among the urban elderly. *Journal of Applied Gerontology*, 2 (June), 216–27.

MacManus, Susan A. (1996a). Young v. old: Campaigns and candidates. *Madison Review* (forthcoming).

———. (1996b). *Young vs. Old: Generational Combat in the 21st Century*. Boulder, CO: Westview Press.

———. (1996c). The widening gap betwen Florida's public schools and their communities: Taxes and a changing age profile. *James Madison Institute Backgrounder*, Policy Report no. 18, February. Tallahassee, FL: James Madison Institute.

———, and Morehouse, Lawrence. (1995). Race, abortion, and judicial retention: The case of the Florida Supreme Court Chief Justice Leander Shaw. In Matthew Holden Jr. (Ed.), *The Changing Regime: Rigidity within Fluidity. Vol. 5. National Political Science Review*, pp. 133–51. New Jersey: Transaction Books.

McKenzie, Richard B. (1993). Senior power: Has the powr of the elderly peaked? *The American Enterprise*, 4 (May–June), 74–80.

Miles, Anne Daughterty. (1995). Politically Active Senior Citizens: How They Compare with Their Politically Inactive Peers. Paper presented at the Annual Meeting of the Midwest Political Science Association, Chicago, IL.

Peterson, Steven A., and Somit, Albert. (1992). Older women: Health and political behavior. *Women and Politics*, 12(4), 87–108.

———. (1994). *The Political Behavior of Older Americans*. New York: Garland Publishing.

Pratt, Henry J. (1976). *The Gray Lobby*. Chicago: University of Chicago Press.

Rosenstone, Steven J., and Hansen, John Mark. (1993). *Mobilization, Participation, and Democracy in America*. New York: Macmillan.

Shaffer, Stephen D., and Breaux, David. (1992). Generational Differences among Southern Grassroots Party Workes. Paper presented at the 1992 Annual Meeting of the American Political Science Association, Chicago, IL, 3–6 September.

Steckenrider, Janie S., and Cutler, Neal E. (1989). Aging and adult political socialization. In R. Siegel (Ed.), *Political Learning in Adulthood*, pp. 56–88. Chicago: University of Chicago Press.

Straits, Bruce C. (1990). The social context of voter turnout. *Public Opinion Quarterly*, 54(1), 64–73.

Strate, John M., Parrish, Charles J., Elder, Charles D., and Ford, III, Coit. (1989). Life span civic development and voting participation. *American Political Science Review*, 83, 443–64.

Texeira, Ruy A. (1992). *The Disappearing American Voter*. Washington, DC: Brookings Institution.

Times Mirror Center for The People and The Press. (1992). *The People, The Press, and Politics, Campaign '92: The Generations Divide*. Washington, DC: Times Mirror for the People and the Press.

U.S. Bureau of the Census. (1992). *Sixty-Five Plus in America*. Current Population Reports, Series P–25, no. 1092. Washington, DC: U.S. Government Printing Office.

Chapter 8 *Re-read*

Old-Age Interest Groups in the 1990s: Coalition, Competition, and Strategy

CHRISTINE L. DAY

During the last three decades, the rise in number, size, diversity, and visibility of political organizations representing older Americans has been phenomenal. The "gray lobby" (Pratt, 1976) had developed a great deal of influence and respect within Washington policy circles by the 1980s. At the same time, the consensus surrounding government old-age programs and benefits had begun to crack (Day, 1990; Hudson, 1978). Older people, previously stereotyped as the deserving poor, were now often blamed for consuming an increasingly burdensome portion of the federal budget (Binstock, 1983). Arguments that older people were receiving more than their "fair share" of government benefits were often framed in terms of "generational equity" (Torres-Gil, 1992; see chapter by Rhodebeck in this volume). These developments began to challenge the legitimacy and influence of old-age interest groups.

The challenge persists in the 1990s, but less as a result of generational conflict, and more as a result of ideological polarization. By the early 1990s, the politics of aging was becoming entangled in the ideological conflicts sweeping American politics in general. This growing ideological polarization arose from a variety of sources. First, a series of social movements in the 1960s and 1970s—including the civil rights, women's rights, and environmental and consumer safety movements—challenged the status quo; interest groups that emerged from these movements have yielded at least some countervailing power to entrenched business and economic interests (Berry, 1984; McFarland, 1987). Second, as the number and variety of interest groups expanded, the resources available to government to meet group demands began to contract, casualties of slower economic growth, persistent federal deficits, and gradually, public rebellion against taxes. Third, and partly as a result of the second, the federal government became increasingly centralized, as partisan battles over the budget replaced decentralized funding of programs favoring a variety of interests (Peterson, 1992). Finally, technological developments, and changes in campaign finance laws requiring fundraising from large numbers of small contributors, led to massive grassroots mobilization efforts, particularly by computerized direct mail. Such efforts are often driven by extreme, simplistic appeals to captivate people's attention and support (Cigler and Loomis, 1995; Godwin, 1988).

A major difference between the current ideological realignment and those of earlier modern times—for example, the rise of the New Deal coalition and Great Society/War on Poverty commitments to greater social, economic, and political equality—is that prior debates were between those who favored the status quo and those who supported greater government efforts in social welfare and equality. Today, the debate is primarily between those who wish, at a minimum, to maintain the status quo, and those who are committed to reducing the role of government in those areas. This may intensify the conflict, as people tend to be more fervent in defense of what they already have than in efforts to achieve something new (Quattrone and Tversky, 1988).

Until recently, most major government programs benefiting the elderly have escaped major cuts, and the elderly have fared better than many other groups. But with Social Security and Medicare alone consuming nearly a third of the federal budget, it is inevitable that these and other age-related programs are now, or likely soon to be, on the congressional chopping block. Congressional staffers interviewed in 1995[1] cited the Medicare Catastrophic Coverage Act (MCCA) of 1988 as the watershed event that swept popular old-age programs, especially Medicare, into the ideological maelstrom. Previously, a bipartisan consensus protected Medicare from major reductions. After a ground swell of protest against raising some older people's taxes in order to pay for Medicare expansion forced the repeal of most MCCA provisions in 1989, conservatives in government perceived new opportunities to justify further cutbacks in the name of smaller government and lower taxes.

How have aging-based political organizations reacted to these changes in the political environment? This chapter, based primarily on interviews with interest group leaders and a few congressional staff members, examines their reactions in terms of organizational origin and maintenance, political strategy and decision making, and patterns of coalition and competition among interest groups.

Interest Group Origin and Maintenance

Aging-oriented interest groups proliferated and diversified during the 1970s and 1980s. The groups ranged in breadth from the all-encompassing American Association of Retired Persons (AARP) to organizations representing ethnic, gender, occupational, and low-income subgroups. They varied in their target memberships from professionals and practitioners to mass memberships. Their structures ranged from large networks of local chapters to direct-mail and staff organizations based entirely in Washington, D.C. And they covered the ideological spectrum from right to left.

Theories of Origin and Maintenance

Where did all of these groups come from? Truman's classic pluralist theory of interest group formation and maintenance (1951) suggests that organizations naturally form as a result of disturbances or threats to a group's well-being. However, Walker (1983) noted that most old-age political organizations were not founded until after the establishment of major programs benefiting the aging such as Medicare, Medicaid, and the Older Americans Act, and the substantial expansion of Social Security benefits. Organizations that did exist became more politicized, as well, after those gains had been achieved. Walker emphasized the role of patronage by such institutions as government, corporations, and private foundations in the origin and maintenance of political organizations. Furthermore, the creation and expansion of government benefits produce new groups of people who have a stake in government programs and who are especially receptive to organizational appeals in defense of those programs (Pratt, 1993). Thus government actions are often a cause, and not just a consequence, of organizational formation and maintenance.

The state-centered approach goes a long way toward explaining developments in the origin and evolution of aging-based interest groups. The evolution of three of the largest mass membership groups illustrates this (Day, 1990; Pratt, 1993; Van Tassel and Meyer, 1992). AARP was originally a service-oriented organization founded in 1947 with the purpose of providing easily available, low-cost insurance to retirees; its large-scale political activities developed years later with the growth of federal aging and retirement programs. The National Council of Senior Citizens (NCSC) has been politically active from the beginning; it was founded in 1961 by leaders of labor unions and Senior Citizens for Kennedy with the purpose of pushing for passage of Medicare. Originally two-thirds of its funding came from union contributions and from the Democratic National Committee; by the 1990s, restricted grants from the federal government comprised over 90% of its revenue, apart from its political action committee.[2] The National Committee to Preserve Social Security and Medicare (NCPSSM), like many political organizations founded in recent years, began in 1982 as a direct-mail organization urging recipients of its mailings to contact public officials and to become dues-paying organization members. Within a few years it had achieved massive letter-writing campaigns and petitions to Congress and a membership in the millions. Yet its long-term survival was rather tenuous because of its negative reputation with the government; many officials criticized the "scare tactics" used in its mailings and its superficial dealings with Congress. Over the next several years, the NCPSSM developed a professional research and lobbying capacity, created a political action committee, and hired a number of prominent officials including its current president, former Social Security Commissioner Martha McSteen. These actions have considerably enhanced the NCPSSM's legitimacy with public officials.

Another challenge to Truman's (1951) "disturbance theory" of interest group formation and maintenance came from Olson (1965), who posited that threats to a group's well-being were not sufficient to entice people to organize. Rational persons know they can "free ride," or benefit from an interest group's accomplishments even if they do not join the group. The exchange theory of interest group origin and maintenance, arising from Olson's work, proposes that interest group leaders overcome the free rider problem and entice members to join with three types of incentives: material incentives, or products with monetary value; solidary incentives, or opportunities to meet and befriend others with common interests; and purposive incentives, or the satisfaction of actively supporting an important cause (Clark and Wilson, 1961; Salisbury, 1969).

Aging-based membership groups use a variety of incentives to attract and retain members (Day, 1990). AARP is well-known for its material incentives, including low-cost insurance, mail-order pharmaceuticals and other discounts, investment opportunities, publications, and a wide array of other products and services that have attracted an astronomical 33 million members. Other groups offer similar products, but not on a scale with AARP. Some groups, including the NCSC, Gray Panthers, the Older Women's League (OWL), and the National Association of Retired Federal Employees (NARFE), combine solidary and purposive incentives in encouraging members to join and participate in local chapters and networks throughout the country; the NARFE, in fact, has required its members to join local chapters since 1986. AARP has 4,000 local chapters, but most are more social than political in nature, and only about 3% of its members belong to them; in addition, around 250,000 AARP members are trained as political and service volunteers. Some groups, like the NCPSSM, use computerized direct mail to offer purposive incentives of the "checkbook" variety (Hayes, 1983): by mailing in their dues and perhaps writing letters or signing postcards or petitions to lawmakers, members can support a cause at relatively low cost in terms of money and time.

The Expansion of Direct-Mail Organizations

Pratt (1993) describes "an apparent saturation" of age-related interest groups in national politics by the late 1980s. Yet in the midnineties, those groups all survive and at least three more have been added to the landscape. Three new groups, Seniors Coalition, the United Seniors Association (USA), and the 60/Plus Association, joined the National Alliance of Senior Citizens (NASC) at the conservative end of the spectrum (Serafini, 1995). The three new organizations, as well as the NASC, support limited government in the area of social welfare, free market reforms and partial or full privatization of old-age benefits, and in general, the provisions of the Republican "Contract With America." But while the NASC, founded twenty years ago, is largely an educational and fund-raising direct-mail organization that has always kept a low profile on Capitol Hill, the three new groups have developed a visible presence in Washington.

All three began between 1989 and 1992 as direct-mail fund-raising organizations with the help of right-wing direct-mail pioneer

Richard Viguerie, who still handles mailings for the USA and 60/Plus. This has opened up the groups to the same types of criticism faced by the NCPSSM when it began as a direct-mail organization ten years ago: that the groups are more interested in making money than in working to influence policy. But like the NCPSSM before them, these groups have enhanced their research and lobbying capacity and their relationships with policymakers. Some Republican Hill staffers claim that the groups, Seniors Coalition and the USA in particular, are now among the most visible and most useful lobbyists for old-age interests, and many conservative members of Congress are delighted to report that (some) senior organizations support their proposals. Representatives from the three groups have, not surprisingly, been invited many times to testify on Capitol Hill since the Republicans gained a congressional majority in 1994. Critics, including representatives of the more liberal aging organizations and Democrats in Congress, counter that the three organizations are being used by conservative lawmakers rather than exerting real influence. But the groups' increased visibility since the 1994 elections is one more example of the symbiotic relationship between interest groups and policymakers described by Pratt in his state-centered approach (1993).

Like the NCPSSM and other direct-mail organizations, the incentives that these new groups offer to members are largely purposive: pay your dues; write to Congress; support the cause. In this way, the three claim to have memberships of several hundred thousand, or two million in the case of Seniors Coalition. What is the leaders' primary motivation? Sabatier (1992) distinguishes between the exchange theory and the commitment theory of interest group formation. Both theories stress the importance of membership incentives offered by group leaders. Exchange theory, however, emphasizes the entrepreneurial nature of interest group leaders who are most interested in their own personal gain. Commitment theory, in contrast, emphasizes leaders' strong commitment to collective political goals. Naturally, leaders of Seniors Coalition, the USA, and 60/Plus stress their commitment to achieving conservative, market-oriented political reform, while their critics charge that the group leaders are in it for the money. The USA, in particular, has taken steps to move beyond its direct-mail fund-raising image, establishing a dozen state-level chapters, laying the groundwork for creating a political action committee, and producing a weekly cable show on National Empowerment Television. Time will tell whether the new groups evolve further toward establishing a reputation as full-fledged independent political organizations.

Political Strategy and Mobilization

Today's political environment requires that aging-based interest groups participate in redistributive politics—debates over sweeping changes in broad-based, high-cost programs that substantially redistribute resources from some groups to others (Lowi, 1964). Until now, these groups have been involved more often in the realm of distributive and regulatory policies—for example, incremental changes in Social Security and Medicare, funding for relatively small-scale programs under the Older Americans Act, and consumer protection. Previously, most of their work in redistributive policy involved pushing for new programs such as long-term care coverage, rather than defending existing ones. Now they are faced with serious proposals to reform and reduce Medicare and Medicaid on a grand scale; nonincremental proposed reforms to Social Security are certain to follow.

Two types of logical responses by old-age interest groups to this situation might be, first, to make all-out efforts to mobilize the grassroots on a large scale and, second, to broaden the scope of issues on the organizational agenda. Mobilizing widespread grassroots participation not only raises political awareness and demonstrates intense public support, but also aids in fund-raising to subsidize other lobbying efforts. Broadening the scope of important issues creates opportunities for an organization to forge broader coalitions and to get involved in politics at a higher level of ideological debate. Interest groups that fail to do so often get lost in the realm of redistributive politics where political parties and top government officials dominate the game (Peterson, 1992; Ripley and Franklin, 1991). Neither of these responses is easy, however, as characteristics of interest group politics mitigate against both increasing grassroots involvement and expanding a group's agenda.

Mobilizing the Grassroots

Grassroots lobbying and mobilization have, in general, become increasingly important in national interest group politics, often eclipsing the more traditional direct lobbying tactics (Cigler and Loomis, 1995). Indeed, congressional staff interviewees contend that large-scale grassroots mobilization at the district or state level, demonstrating the electoral importance of an issue, is more important than monetary contributions, especially for redistributive policy; the broader the issue, one noted, the more important the grassroots pressure and the less important the PAC contributions. This is especially true for old-age mass membership groups. Many policymakers acknowledge the importance of some aging groups' research and information sharing through direct lobbying, and through other groups' PAC contributions, but these mass membership organizations are most prominent on Capitol Hill for their grassroots mobilization. They are among the most successful of all political organizations in flooding Congress with mail and phone calls (Cook and Barrett, 1992; Day, 1990; Fowler and Shaiko, 1987). And many still recall the image of older people surrounding Rep. Dan Rostenkowski's car in protest against the Medicare Catastrophic Coverage Act of 1988.

If aging-based groups are increasing their grassroots and other resource mobilization efforts, however, it appears to be more a long-term trend than a reaction to recent events. AARP, for example, evolved from a largely service-oriented group to a prominent advocacy organization, increasing its political direct-mail efforts and establishing AARP/VOTE, a voter education program that publishes candidates' stands on issues, in the mid-1980s. More recent AARP efforts are aimed at building up its state and local offices and chapters (U.S. Congress, 1995:97). Other groups such as the National Council of Senior Citizens (NCSC) and Families U.S.A. increased their direct mail operations in the 1980s and 1990s; still others, like the National Committee to Preserve Social Security and Medicare, (NCPSSM), Seniors Coalition, and the United Seniors Association (USA), supplemented highly successful direct-mail operations with expanded lobbying efforts to increase their legitimacy on Capitol Hill. Groups such as the Gray Panthers and the Older Women's League (OWL), which always emphasized organizing at the local level, moved their headquarters to Washington, D.C., in the 1980s and partially centralized their structures in order to better coordinate local activities. The National Association of Retired Federal Employees (NARFE) hoped to increase district-level activity and pressure on public officials by requiring members to join local chapters beginning in 1986. Several interviewees referred to one particularly recent trend common to several of these organizations: the attempt to increase organization efforts at the state, local, and district levels. This is, perhaps, a logical reaction to serious congressional proposals to redistribute policy responsibilities to the states (Liebig, 1992).

Mobilizing members to action, whether through local networks or mass communications, requires a large infusion of resources, and therefore is easier said than done. In addition, increasing membership involvement in organizational activity and decision making poses a dilemma for organization leaders. While a high degree of member involvement may increase an organization's legitimacy in the eyes of both members and public officials, it also decreases the control that leaders exert over the organization (McCarthy and Zald, 1977).

Three Types of Mobilization

In terms of member participation and mobilization, there are at least three organizational types, each with its own dilemmas (see Table 8.1). First are the organizations that rely on solidary and purposive incentives to encourage member involvement at the local chapter level, working together face-to-face. These include NARFE, OWL, NCSC, and the Gray Panthers. Since such activities require intense commitments of time and energy, relatively few members are likely to respond. As Gray Panthers founder Maggie Kuhn (1976:91) put it, ". . . we cannot hope to motivate everybody over 65. . . . We have modest goals and hopes for the enlistment of small numbers of wrinkled radicals who are fully committed people. . . . " Their active members may indeed be committed, but these are not the organizations that enjoy the highest degree of visibility and influence in government, at least not on broad redistributive policy. NARFE is quite successful in the relatively narrow range of issues directly affecting federal retirees; the NCSC maintains strong and beneficial ties to the broader labor movement and Democratic officials; leaders of the OWL and the Gray Panthers maintain connections and a good deal of respect among many high officials. But seldom, if ever, do policymakers list these organizations among the most significant in aging policy circles.

The second organizational type is one that relies on purposive incentives, relayed through mass communications such as direct mail, to engage large numbers of people at a relatively low level of commitment. These include the NCPSSM, the USA, and the Seniors Coalition. Their visibility on Capitol Hill is high but their influence is problematic. Members of Congress and their staff often are irritated by the mountains of mail generated by direct-mail organizations, likening their grassroots to Astroturf; at the same time, they acknowledge that such tactics are difficult to ignore and may affect policy (Cigler and Loomis, 1995; Day, 1990).

Finally, there are the organizations that rely substantially on material incentives to attract mass memberships with varying

Table 8.1
Membership Incentives and Mobilization

Incentive Type	Solidary/Purposive	Purposive Only	Material
Commitment Required:	Intense; Much Time and Energy	Low Level	Varying
Level of Mobilization:	Local Chapter	National Organization of Individuals	National; Moderate Local Chapter Activity
Interaction Type:	Face-to-Face	Mass Communication Direct Mail	Varying
Examples:	NARFE, NCSC, OWL, Gray Panthers	NCPSSM, USA, Seniors Coalition	AARP

degrees of commitment to the organization's political goals; the 33-million member AARP is the quintessential example. AARP is without question the most ubiquitous and powerful "800-pound gorilla" among aging-based organizations. However, attempting to represent such a large and diverse membership leads to problems in both the organization's internal and external relations. Internally, the leadership's issue positions may generate active and angry dissent among millions of members, even if leaders contend that most members agree with the leadership. This occurred at least twice in recent years, when many AARP members protested against AARP's support for the Medicare Catastrophic Act (MCCA) of 1988 and for Democratic leaders' health care reform proposals in the early 1990s (Crystal, 1990; Day, 1993; *New York Times*, 1994).

Externally, the attempt to represent a massive and diverse membership opens the organization to criticism from all sides, especially in times of broad ideological conflict. Whereas ten years ago public officials often portrayed AARP as the voice of moderation, widely informative, and easy to work with (Day, 1990), that type of assessment is much less common today. Liberal policymakers and leaders of liberal organizations contend that AARP represents primarily its wealthier and more privileged members. Indeed, this is not uncommon among mass membership organizations of all types, as the more vocal, active, and politically aware members tend to come from the middle and upper classes (Moe, 1980); AARP leaders acknowledge the same tendencies. At the same time, conservative officials and leaders of conservative organizations fault AARP for representing only their liberal Democratic members, and justify their criticism by pointing to the MCCA and health care reform controversies.

Organizational Diversity and Issue Specialization

Expanding an organization's issue agenda, like mobilizing its constituency, is difficult and problematic for organization leaders. Interest groups are generally more successful when their policy goals are narrow and specific than when they are broad in scope (Ripley and Franklin, 1991; Schlozman and Tierney, 1986). Leaders of the NARFE, for example, maintain that one of the secrets of their success—in addition to a politically savvy constituency, retired federal employees—is their narrow primary focus on defending the uniqueness of federal retirement benefits. More generally, old-age interest groups have been most successful when defending relatively small-scale programs, or when defending against incremental changes in large programs (Binstock, 1972, 1990; Day, 1990; Heclo, 1988; Wallace and Williamson, 1992).

Furthermore, several interest group leaders noted one of the ironies of the current political environment: With many social welfare and related benefits under broad ideological attack, many interest groups recognize the value of presenting a united front in their defense. Yet this defensive stance requires each group to focus intensely on its own specific interests, hoping that others will take care of their own; thus active coalitions are discouraged.

Browne's (1990) research on organizational agenda setting and interaction in the agricultural policy domain uncovered a pattern of narrow issue orientation and avoidance of intense alliances or adversarial relationships. Rather, interest groups tend to specialize in a small range of issues and to market themselves as such within their issue networks. Some groups are broader in purpose than others, but each develops its own issue niche, resulting in a kind of "plural elitism."

Aging-based interest groups demonstrate the same tendency to develop their own niches and to recognize each other's relatively exclusive roles. The process of group self-definition and mutual recognition appears to evolve over time. The NCSC, to take one example, has always maintained ties to the labor movement in its advocacy and organization, but more recently invests much of its effort in helping to administer federally sponsored low-income employment and other programs. Aging-based groups focusing on ethnic and racial minorities engage in similar activities through government contracts, but primarily for their narrower constituencies.

The Families USA Foundation, established in 1981 to advocate for the elderly poor, has narrowed its issue focus almost exclusively to health care, particularly Medicaid and long-term care. The National Council on the Aging likewise has become more involved in health care reform "than in any other issue ever," according to a representative. The Gray Panthers has always had a broad intergenerational and peace-oriented agenda, but in recent years has focused most of its resources on the three issues of campaign reform, jobs and full employment, and universal health care coverage. The OWL's niche lies naturally at the intersection of aging and women's interests, focusing on older women's health care and income security needs as well as such gender-specific issues as workplace discrimination and domestic violence. The NCPSSM has, over time, established its own niche in battling changes that would reduce any aspect of Social Security and Medicare benefits or raise older people's taxes to pay for those benefits. Often shunned by other aging-based organizations in the past because of its extremism and exclusive direct-mail approach, the NCPSSM is now much more accepted in its particular role. AARP's broad agenda and diverse constituency seems to transcend any narrowly specialized issue niche, but AARP is selective in its issue priorities at any given time and cautious about selecting priorities that might stir up opposition within subgroups of its diverse constituency.

In sum, while developments in the political environment might push old-age organizations toward a more broad-based ideological agenda, the trend among individual groups is more often in the opposite direction: toward a more narrow and exclusive issue orientation mutually respected by the other groups. The exceptions currently are the three new conservative organizations, Seniors Coalition, the USA, and 60/Plus, which appear to be competing for the same niche. They may not criticize each other publicly, but interestingly, they also do not appear to be working closely together, despite sharing nearly identical origins and goals. If they all survive in the long term, they will likely evolve along different paths until they diverge sufficiently from each other and establish their own distinct political specialties. Just as business entrepreneurs must differentiate their products from others in order to gain a significant market share, so must interest group entrepreneurs differentiate their organizations from others in order to attract and maintain significant memberships. Should the three new conservative old-age groups fail to establish distinct organizational identities, one is likely eventually to drive the other two out of the market.

Coalitions, Strategic Alliances, and Adversarial Relations

In the pluralistic world of interest group politics, building broad coalitions can be as difficult as building a broader issue agenda. Aging-based political organizations face myriad conflicting motives both to engage in broad-based coalition building and to eschew such coalitions for more narrow, transitory, and fragmented intergroup interactions. The broad conservative movement to alter the role of government, balance the budget, and turn back social policy responsibilities to the states confronts old-age organizations with the need to form a united front with other groups interested in preserving social programs. But coalition building is costly in terms of group autonomy and the ability to claim exclusive credit for group achievements (Day, 1990). Coalition building is also difficult when group benefits are threatened, according to organization leaders; each group becomes concerned with defending its own specific interests.

Patterns of Coalition Building

Empirical examination of group conflict and coalition in various domains (Heinz, et al., 1993) shows group interaction patterns to be fragmented and lacking in central coordination or mediation. The exception is the labor policy domain, in which peak associations of labor and business engage in more encompassing ideological conflict. A peak association is one that dominates within a policy area, such as the AFL-CIO within the labor domain, or the U.S. Chamber of Commerce and the National Association of Manufacturers within the business sector (ibid.). There is no peak association among aging-based groups; even AARP does not span the interests of narrower aging-based groups and speak collectively for the entire sector. Furthermore, consumer groups (e.g., those of the aging), even more than producer groups, operate in a wide variety of issue networks and tend to form coalitions that are fragmented and temporary (Bykerk and Maney, 1995).

Among old-age interest groups, there appears to be a growing tension between broad coalition building across age groups and a more fragmented special-interest orientation. All of the group representatives interviewed were asked about their major allies and adversaries—or at least groups which, if not direct adversaries, worked against their major interests. Alliances tend to be fragmentary and, as emphasized by virtually all groups, dependent upon the particular issue—a characteristic of American interest group coalitions generally (Gais, Peterson, and Walker, 1984). Aging organizations listed a variety of consumer, children's, women's, labor, public interest, ideological, and other aging-based groups as allies. On some issues, particularly those involving health care, aging groups forge alliances with health care and service provider organizations that often are their adversaries. Organizations representing doctors, hospitals, and nursing homes often clash with elderly groups over issues of government regulation and cost containment, but all have a stake in preserving or expanding government funding of Medicare and Medicaid. AARP, the American Medical Association, and the AFL-CIO, for example, joined forces in 1994 to advertise their support for universal health care coverage and patient choice among doctors and plans (Cigler and Loomis, 1995). The only aging groups that did not cite an array of special interest groups as allies were the conservative organizations—the NASC, Seniors Coalition, and the USA; they named only broadly ideological organizations and think tanks. There is little or no evidence that these conservative aging advocacy organizations work in coalition with other political organizations; rather they seem to share ideas and ideological affinities.

Group representatives were also asked about the importance of horizontal alliances with other aging organizations, and vertical alliances with nonelderly groups (Torres-Gil, 1992). Most said that vertical alliances generally were more important. However, most also indicated that the Leadership Council of Aging Organizations (LCAO), founded in 1978, has proven more valuable and relevant on most issues than Generations United (GU), a coalition of old-age and children's advocacy groups formed in 1986. GU has been a valuable information clearinghouse and forum for discussion, but evidently has not been very active on broad-based issues. The LCAO's importance has grown in the face of threats to elderly programs and benefits, and even the NCPSSM, blackballed for years because of its direct-mail fund raising reputation, was admitted to the LCAO in 1995 because, in the words of one organizational representative, "we need all the friends we can get." Yet the aging-based membership organizations in the LCAO have clashed among themselves on a number of important issues, including the Medicare Catastrophic Coverage Act, and in 1994 they could not agree on which basic principles of health care reform to support (Liebig, 1994).

Adversarial Relations among Organizations

While the patterns of alliances indicate some ideological as well as interest-group pluralist orientation, broad ideological conflict is much more conspicuous in the adversarial relations. Nearly all the aging-based groups listed as their adversaries only broadly ideological conservative organizations and think tanks such as the Heritage Foundation and the Cato Institute, balanced budget advocates such as the Concord Coalition, and business and corporate interests. The conservative aging organizations named AARP as their principal adversary, and their publications abound in criticisms of AARP and, secondarily, the NCSC. The conflicts are clearly more ideological than intergenerational, even though some organizations promoting conservative causes and budget-balancing frame some of their arguments in the language of generational conflict.[3]

Most of the congressional staff members interviewed also perceived the aging organizations' patterns of coalition and competition in ideological terms. Congressional hearings in the last few years have targeted aging organizations according to partisan positions or ideological views. House Democrats in 1992 held hearings to examine allegedly deceptive direct mailings from groups including the Seniors Coalition and the USA (U.S. Congress, 1992). Three years later, Senate Republicans held hearings to examine AARP's business practices and tax-exempt status (U.S. Congress, 1995). Yet despite the partisan nature of congressional-interest group interactions, all aging-based political organizations steadfastly maintain their official nonpartisan status as well as their fragmentary alliances.

Conclusion

Old-age interest groups face several dilemmas in a political environment driven by ideological polarization over the government's social welfare role. Their symbiotic relationships with government and their successful employment of membership incentives seem to assure their long-term survival. But their influence on policy, in the redistributive realm, is problematic without sufficient grassroots commitment and broad coalitional support. Their political strength often lies in grassroots mobilization. But mobilizing a constituency as diverse as older Americans, whether through local networking, direct mail, or mass marketing of services, often leads to internal dissent or charges of manipulation through extreme and simplistic appeals. Their attempts to forge broad coalitions run counter to all interest groups' tendencies toward narrow specialization. Coalition building is even more difficult among groups whose benefits are threatened and who must therefore concentrate on defending their own interests. The result is an increasing tension between traditional, narrow, pluralistic politics and the more difficult but potentially more fruitful efforts toward partisan and ideological unity. In sum, while most of these organizations will surely survive over the long term, their influence on policy will depend on whether they can maintain distinct organizational identities while also expanding their joint efforts with ideologically like-minded groups.

Notes

1. Leaders or staff members who deal with political matters in the following organizations were interviewed during the summer of 1995 (usually one person per organization, occasionally two or three): the American Association of Homes and Services for the Aging, the American Association of Retired Persons, the American Health Care Association, the Concord Coalition, Families U.S.A. Foundation, Generations United, the Gray Panthers, the National AFL-CIO COPE Retiree Program, the National Alliance of Senior Citizens. the National Association of Retired Federal Employees, the National Committee to Preserve Social Security and Medicare, the National Council on the Aging, the National Council of Senior Citizens, the Older Women's League, Seniors Coalition, and the United Seniors Association. The main focus here is on mass membership groups that deal primarily with aging issues and cater to a primarily elderly constituency, although the interviews included a few other aging-related organizations as well. (See Van Tassel and Meyer [1992] for institutional profiles of eighty-three U.S. aging policy interest groups.) In addition, eleven staff members of congressional committees dealing extensively with aging-related policies were interviewed; they included staff from both parties and both chambers of Congress. All interviewees were promised anonymity.

2. Other organizations, including those focused on the needs of racial and ethnic subgroups of older people such as the National Caucus and

Center on Black Aged and the Asociacion Nacional Pro Personal Mayores, also received 90% or more of their funding from the federal government, further illustrating the importance of government patronage to organizational maintenance (see Van Tassel and Meyer, 1992).

3. The same kind of ideological conflict can be seen among young-adult groups, as illustrated by Pramas's article (1995) in *As We Are*, "the magazine for working young people," which disparages the organization Lead or Leave as a corporate-funded right-wing organization posing as an advocate for young people.

References

American Association of Retired Persons (AARP). (1995). *Statement Before the Senate Finance Committee's Subcommittee on Social Security and Family Policy.* 20 June.

Berry, Jeffrey M. (1984). *The Interest Group Society.* Boston: Little, Brown.

Binstock, Robert H. (1972). Interest-group liberalism and the politics of aging. *Gerontologist,* 12, 265–80.

———. (1983). The aged as scapegoat. *Gerontologist,* 23, 136–43.

———. (1990). The politics and economics of aging and diversity. In S. A. Bass, E. G. Kutza, and F. M. Torres-Gil (Eds.), *Diversity in Aging: Challenges Facing Planners and Policymakers in the 1990s.* Glenview, IL: Scott, Foresman.

Browne, William P. (1990). Organized interests and their issue niches: A search for pluralism in a policy domain. *Journal of Politics,* 52, 477–509.

Bykerk, Loree, and Maney, Ardith. (1995). Consumer groups and coalition politics on Capitol Hill. In A. J. Cigler and B. A. Loomis (Eds.), *Interest Group Politics.* 4th ed. Washington, DC: Congressional Quarterly Press.

Cigler, Allan J., and Loomis, Burdett A. (1995). Contemporary interest group politics: More than "More of the Same." In A. J. Cigler and B. A. Loomis (Eds.), *Interest Group Politics.* 4th ed. Washington, DC: Congressional Quarterly Press.

Clark, Peter B., and Wilson, James Q. (1961). Incentive systems: A theory of organizations. *Administrative Science Quarterly,* 6, 219–66.

Cook, Fay Lomax, and Barrett, Edith J. (1992). *Support for the American Welfare State.* New York: Columbia University Press.

Crystal, Stephen. (1990). Health economics, old-age politics, and the Catastrophic Medicare Debate. *Journal of Gerontological Social Work*, 15
(3/4), 21–31.

Day, Christine L. (1990). *What Older Americans Think: Interest Groups
and Aging Policy*. Princeton: Princeton University Press.

————. 1993. Older Americans' attitudes toward the Medicare Catastrophic
Coverage Act of 1988. *Journal of Politics*, 55, 167–77.

Fowler, Linda L., and Shaiko, Ronald G. (1987). The Graying of the Constituency: Active Seniors in Congressional District Politics. Presented
at the annual meeting of the American Political Science Association,
Chicago.

Gais, Thomas L., Peterson, Mark A., and Walker, Jack L. (1984). Interest
groups, iron triangles, and representative institutions in American
national government. *British Journal of Political Science*, 14, 161–
85.

Godwin, R. Kenneth. (1988). *The Direct Marketing of Politics: $1 Billion of
Influence*. Chatham, NJ: Chatham House.

Hayes, Michael T. (1983). Interest groups: Pluralism or mass society? In
J. A. Cigler and B. A. Loomis (Eds.), *Interest Group Politics*. Washington, DC: Congressional Quarterly Press.

Heclo, Hugh. (1988). Generational politics. In J. L. Palmer, T. Smeeding,
and B. Boyle Torrey (Eds.), *The Vulnerable*. Washington, DC: Urban
Institute Press.

Heinz, John P., Laumann, Edward O., Nelson, Robert L., and Salisbury,
Robert H. (1993). *The Hollow Core: Private Interests in National
Policy Making*. Cambridge: Harvard University Press.

Hudson, Robert B. (1978). Emerging pressures on public policies for the
aging. *Society*, 15 (July/August), 30–33.

Kuhn, Margaret E. (1976). What old people want for themselves and others in society. In Paul Kerschner (Ed.), *Advocacy and Age*. Los
Angeles: Ethel Percy Andrus Gerontology Center, University of Southern California.

Liebig, Phoebe S. (1992). Federalism and aging policy in the 1980s: Implications for changing interest group roles in the 1990s. *Journal of
Aging and Social Policy*, 4(1/2), 17–33.

————. (1994). The Aging Coalition, Advocacy and Health Care Reform.
Presented at the annual meeting of the Gerontological Society of
America, Atlanta.

Lowi, Theodore J. (1964). American business, public policy, and political theory. *World Politics*, 16, 677–715.

McCarthy, John D., and Zald, Meyer D. (1977). Resource mobilization and social movements: A partial theory. *American Journal of Sociology*, 82, 1212–41.

McFarland, Andrew S. (1987). Interest groups and theories of power in America. *British Journal of Political Science*, 17, 129–47.

Moe, Terry M. (1980). *The Organization of Interests*. Chicago: University of Chicago Press. *New York Times*. (1994). 17 August, p. 7.

Olson, Mancur Jr. (1965). *The Logic of Collective Action*. Cambridge: Harvard University Press.

Peterson, Paul E. (1992). The rise and fall of special interest politics. In M. P. Petracca (Ed.), *The Politics of Interests: Interest Groups Transformed*. Boulder: Westview Press.

Pramas, Jason. (1995). Lead . . . or leave and the sellout of my generation. *As We Are*, 3 (spring), 27–40 passim.

Pratt, Henry J. (1976). *The Gray Lobby*. Chicago: University of Chicago Press.

———. (1993). *Gray Agendas: Interest Groups and Public Pensions in Canada, Britain, and the United States*. Ann Arbor: University of Michigan Press.

Quattrone, George A., and Tversky, Amos. (1988). Contrasting rational and psychological analyses of political choice. *American Political Science Review*, 82, 719–36.

Ripley, Randall B., and Franklin, Grace A. (1991). *Congress, the Bureaucracy, and Public Policy*. 5th ed. Pacific Grove, CA: Brooks/Cole.

Sabatier, Paul A. (1992). Interest group membership and organization: Multiple theories. In M. P. Petracca (Ed.), *The Politics of Interests: Interest Groups Transformed*. Boulder: Westview Press.

Salisbury, Robert H. (1969). An exchange theory of interest groups. *Midwest Journal of Political Science*, 13, 1–32.

Schlozman, Kay Lehman, and Tierney, John T. (1986). *Organized Interests and American Democracy*. New York: Harper.

Serafini, Marilyn Werber. (1995). Senior schism. *National Journal*, 6 May, pp. 1089–93.

Torres-Gil, Fernando M. (1992). *The New Aging: Politics and Change in America*. New York: Auburn House.

Truman, David B. (1951). *The Governmental Process*. New York: Knopf.

U.S. Congress. (1992). House Committee on Ways and Means, Subcommittees on Oversight and Social Security. *Deceptive Mailings and Solicitations to Senior Citizens and Other Citizens: Hearings*. 102d Cong., 2d sess., 14 May.

————. (1995). Senate Committee on Finance, Subcommittee on Social Security and Family Policy. *Business and Financial Practices of the American Association of Retired Persons: Hearings*. 104th Cong., 1st sess. 13 and 20 June.

Van Tassel, David D., and Meyer, Jimmy Elaine Wilkinson. (1992). *U.S. Aging Policy Interest Groups: Institutional Profiles*. Westport, CT: Greenwood Press.

Walker, Jack L. (1983). The origins and maintenance of interest groups in America. *American Political Science Review*, 77, 390–406.

Wallace, Steven P., and Williamson, John B. (1992). *The Senior Movement: References and Resources*. New York: G. K. Hall.

Chapter 9

Competing Problems, Budget Constraints, and Claims
for Intergenerational Equity

LAURIE A. RHODEBECK

Certain politicians and activists have been raising the issue of intergenerational equity for more than a decade. Broader interest in the issue has developed only recently, perhaps as a consequence of concerns emerging in budgetary politics. Giving particular attention to spending preferences indicative of generational conflict over policy priorities, this study examines public attitudes toward government spending and their relationship to congressional policy-making. I begin by describing the emergence and development of the intergenerational equity issue, then turn to consider it in the context of recent budgetary politics. Budget negotiations provide opportunities to shape public opinion about government spending, thereby heightening or diminishing conflict among groups that stand to win or lose as a result of different funding decisions. I focus specifically on the potential for age group conflict of the sort implied by the intergenerational equity issue. Then, using data on public attitudes toward government spending, I examine age-specific preferences in policy areas at the forefront of recent deliberations over the budget. I also assess the relationship between these preferences and voting behavior in the 1994 congressional election. In concluding, I discuss the link between public opinion and public policy and its implications for the debate over intergenerational equity.

Intergenerational Equity

Contemporary concerns about intergenerational equity arose first among members of the American business community in the early 1970s, apparently in reaction to legislation that amended the Social Security program to provide many new benefits to retirees. When program funding problems developed in the late 1970s and intensified in the early 1980s, business leaders began to voice dire predictions about the viability of the Social Security system and its increasing burden on young workers and taxpayers (Quadagno, 1989).

The equity issue entered the national political arena in 1984, when Sen. David Durenberger (R-MN) and Rep. James Jones (D-OK) founded Americans for Generational Equity (AGE). Funded substantially by private sector alternatives to Social Security and Medicare (e.g., health care corporations, insurance companies, and banks), AGE proposed "to reframe the parameters of the Social Security debate and ultimately alter social policy" (Quadagno, 1989:361). AGE developed a bipartisan appeal and articulated a range of policy concerns, including Medicare reform, savings and investment options, educational priorities, and deficit reduction. Although it failed to achieve any specific policy goals, AGE did succeed in reframing the debate over social benefits for the elderly so that future policy choices would be considered with intergenerational equity in mind. AGE also managed to create the notion that greedy, selfish older people are to blame for the problem of inadequate resources for younger generations. Its message of a generational struggle over scarce resources quickly gained currency in leading newspapers and periodicals,[1] and prominent scholars on its advisory board introduced the intergenerational equity message to academic audiences.[2]

AGE faded from the political scene, but other organizations have taken up its concerns. Most of these groups share the mission of encouraging thrift in government spending. One of the more visible organizations, the Concord Coalition, was founded by former senators Warren Rudman (R-NH) and Paul Tsongas (D-MA) in the wake of the 1992 elections. It aims to eliminate the federal deficit and to educate voters about the rationale for budget cuts. The Concord Coalition avoids pernicious characterizations of the elderly but relentlessly attacks federal entitlement programs for contributing to the deficit (Lacayo, 1993). One of its standard policy proposals is an affluence test on entitlements for retirees, a suggestion the group has reiterated while lobbying for Medicare reform during recent congressional budget deliberations.

Other groups have a broader mission and a more hostile message. Third Millennium stands out among them for its challenge, in both form and substance, to older generations. The group speaks for an age cohort whose senior members are barely 30 years old. Every problem identified by Third Millennium—from the burgeoning national debt to the deteriorating natural environment—is accompanied by a common diagnosis: the self-indulgence of older Americans is to blame (Butterworth, 1993). Although the organization claims it does not want to foster generational conflict, most of its proposals are explicitly touted for their ability to achieve intergenerational equity. Indeed, the group's founding document, the "Third Millennium Declaration" (1993), is an unambiguous expression of backlash against what members perceive are the undeserved benefits enjoyed by the elderly. Acting on their beliefs, members of Third Millennium testified before the first session of the 104th Congress on matters that ranged from the impending insolvency of Medicare to the need to reform Social Security (Thau, 1995). Complaints about the unfairness and unsoundness of current entitlement policies also surfaced among group members attending the 1995 White House Conference on Aging, who left with the feeling that their attempts to seek "generational cooperation" were derailed by partisan politics and the inflexibility of their elders (Strauss and Dee, 1995).

As these examples indicate, policies that benefit the aged are not universally supported by organized political actors. This is not news to older Americans and the organizations that represent them. Advocates for senior citizens have for some time now tried to dispel the impression that resource allocation in an aging society automatically pits the young against the old. They argue that emphasizing the maldistribution of resources between age groups diverts attention from complex structural problems that foster inequality within all age groups (Kingson, 1988). At the grassroots level, commentary in *Modern Maturity*, the bimonthly publication of the American Association of Retired Persons (AARP), increasingly stresses the need for all ages to cooperate in solving social problems. Prior to the 1995 White House Conference on Aging, for example, the executive director of AARP urged that the main issues at the conference—health care, income security, work, and consumer problems—"be approached in the context of generational interdependence" (Deets, 1994).

These conciliatory messages seem to be attempts to remind older Americans to think about the welfare of younger citizens, because until now there has been no reason to persuade young people to support the needs of the elderly. Two decades of survey data indicate that enthusiasm for such programs as Social Security and Medicare has been high among young and old alike. Even a 1994 survey commissioned by Third Millennium failed to reveal the sort of conflict that characterizes elite debate on intergenerational equity (*The Public Perspective,* 1995). Based on this evidence it would be difficult to argue that the issue of intergenerational equity has divided the mass public into conflicting age groups. When citizens disagree about old-age entitlement programs, their divergent views are shaped by partisanship and economics, not age (Day, 1990; Rhodebeck, 1993). Recent politics could, however, alter this picture.

Intergenerational Equity and Budgetary Politics

In 1994, dissatisfaction with business-as-usual, especially the usual Democratic business, contributed to a partisan sea-change in Congress, which in turn has inspired a reexamination of the federal deficit, entitlement programs, and the role of government in providing for the welfare of certain citizens. The "Contract with America," announced by Republicans in the midst of the 1994 congressional elections, promised to address "fiscal responsibility" and "personal responsibility," among other broad issues of growing concern to citizens and their representatives. Upon becoming the majority in Congress, Republican legislators proceeded to keep their promise, first by attempting to pass the balanced budget amendment, then by initiating hearings on welfare reform. Welfare and the budget will certainly remain at the top of the legislative agenda for some time, fueling partisan debates about what government should or should not provide for different citizens and how to fund whatever obligations the federal government does assume.

Congressional Republicans can claim strong public support for their general effort to restore fiscal responsibility: nearly 80% of adult Americans favor a constitutional amendment that would require the federal government to balance its books by 2002 (Berke, 1995). The difficulties arise in finding ways to reduce the deficit on which all can agree. Almost no one expresses enthusiasm for higher taxes. Spending cuts are acceptable to most people, as long as the cuts do not affect programs from which they benefit (MacManus, 1995). Apparently the Republican notion of "personal responsibility" is popular only when it pertains to someone other than oneself. Thus, the problem is what to cut and by how much in order to reach the publicly approved goals of reducing the deficit and eventually balancing the budget, without alienating certain constituencies of voters.

Because the largest and fastest-growing areas of federal spending are entitlement programs, and because Social Security and Medicare account for the biggest shares of entitlement spending (Hager, 1993), the issues of fiscal responsibility, personal responsibility, and intergenerational equity are intertwined. The links among these issues are forged by the reality and the rhetoric of budgetary politics. Three budgetary realities and the rhetoric surrounding them are especially noteworthy.

One reality is that expenditures must be cut if raising taxes is not an option for reducing the deficit. Although some members of Congress have proposed ways to trim Social Security spending, the party line among both Democrats and Republicans is that cuts in this entitlement program are "off the table."[3] This position is unacceptable to anyone concerned with intergenerational equity. By giving Social Security a protected status in the budget, the burden of spending cuts inevitably shifts to other areas, such as education, that affect the welfare of younger generations. The rhetoric associated with the special treatment of Social Security has much to do with the potential for generational conflict over old-age entitlement spending. Legislators can emphasize the need to protect Social Security from the partisan politics of the budget so that future generations of retirees will be able to enjoy the benefits of the program. Alternatively, they can accentuate how current retirees benefit from the program at the expense of younger citizens. Recent discussions of the budget provide examples of both perspectives.

Medicare, in contrast, has been on the front line of budget cuts. For example, during the 1995 budget deliberations, House Republicans proposed to cut approximately $270 billion from Medicare spending over the next seven years, as a major step toward balancing the federal budget. Whether a cut of this magnitude is in reality necessary has been obscured by the rhetoric accompanying the proposal. Aware that Medicare is as important to senior citizens as Social Security, Republican legislators have been careful to speak of "slowing the rate of increase" in Medicare spending instead of using the word "cut." Democrats who oppose reducing

Medicare expenditures invariably use the word and often mention the pain such a cut will inflict on the elderly (Kolbert, 1995).

Public response to the partisan debate indicates that rhetorical efforts to shape the Medicare issue have had mixed success. On the one hand, polls conducted by the Concord Coalition and AARP about two months after the Republicans announced their plans found that a majority of voters believe changes in Medicare are necessary to balance the budget (Broder, 1995). On the other hand, a poll commissioned by the American Hospital Association and conducted by a Republican pollster found that a majority of Americans see Medicare as fundamentally tied to Social Security and consider cuts to Medicare as unacceptable as cuts to Social Security, which people believe legislators, Republican and Democratic, had promised to avoid (Toner, 1995a).

The second reality of budgetary politics is that funds for both Medicare and Social Security will run out in the near future. Projections used in the 1995 budget negotiations estimated that Medicare funds will dry up by 2002, and that Social Security funds will be gone by 2030 (*Social Security Bulletin,* 1995). This situation raises serious questions about what younger generations can expect in the way of public support during their later years. Although legislators generally agree on the nature of the looming problems, differences of opinion over solutions are framed in partisan rhetoric that echoes the debate on reducing Medicare expenditures to balance the budget. Republicans emphasize that "radical restructuring" of Medicare is essential to preserve the program for the next generation (Rubin, 1995), while Democrats charge that the "cuts will devastate seniors for decades" (House Minority Leader Richard A. Gephardt, D-MO, quoted in Fraley, 1995:1900).

The third reality is that reforms to entitlement programs, whether to promote fiscal responsibility or to encourage personal responsibility, are essential. Demographic changes, a sour economy, and rising health care costs have pushed spending on the major entitlement programs to unprecedented levels. Fraud and inefficiency in some programs have contributed to the perception that tighter reins on funds are necessary. Finally, the unintended social consequences of public welfare have led many citizens and their representatives to advocate that the distribution of entitlement benefits be restricted to individuals who meet certain stipulations. Again, Republicans and Democrats agree on the need for reforms (Toner, 1995b), but they tend to frame their proposals in the rhetoric typical of their party (Jacoby, 1995). Perhaps the clearest difference in partisan rhetoric is the tendency for Republicans to focus on general, symbolic appeals (e.g., lower taxes and getting government off our backs), while Democrats emphasize specific, programmatic details (e.g., tax breaks for the middle class and providing assistance to those most in need). Partisanship aside, debate on entitlement reforms is usually carefully phrased to distinguish popular welfare programs that offer social security (e.g., Social Security and Medicare) from less popular welfare programs that offer social assistance (e.g., food stamps and family support). Sweeping attacks on entitlement spending miss this distinction and risk incurring the wrath of electorally active constituencies who benefit from or support social security programs.

Whatever the final choices, the exercise of formulating a budget under the "mandate" of bringing fiscal responsibility to the federal government forces legislators to make difficult choices in an atmosphere of public ambivalence about which programs should be trimmed and the size of the cuts. Legislators worry about making good policy choices. In doing so they have an opportunity to educate the public about the need for, and implications of, certain choices, some of which are sure to be unpopular. But legislators also worry about public response to their policy choices. In anticipating what decisions are likely to be popular, legislators make choices that help assure their reelection. There is, in short, a dynamic relationship between policy-making and public opinion. Three aspects of this relationship are the focus of the following analyses. First, what are the spending priorities of the public in a political climate that stresses fiscal and personal responsibility? Do recent priorities differ from those expressed over the past decade? Second, to what extent do these priorities reflect concerns raised by the intergenerational equity debate? Are there clear age differences in attitudes about policies that have age-specific benefits? Finally, what relationship do these priorities have to congressional politics? Do different spending priorities translate into variations in electoral support that benefit either the Republicans or the Democrats?

Public Attitudes toward Government Spending

The Data

To examine these issues more systematically, data collected by the University of Michigan Center for Political Studies during the past decade is analyzed.[4] Data from the 1994 National Election

Study (NES), is primarily employed and is occasionally supplemented with data from some of their earlier surveys. The surveys include two types of items that measure attitudes toward government spending. One is a general question that asks respondents to indicate where their opinion fits on a seven-point scale anchored at one extreme by the view that "government should provide many fewer services; reduce spending a lot" and at the other extreme by the view that "government should provide many more services; increase spending a lot."[5] The other set of items is introduced by a question that asks respondents, "If you had a say in making up the federal budget this year, for which of the following programs would you like to see spending increased and for which would you like to see spending decreased?" The response categories are "increased," " decreased," and "kept about the same." In 1994 respondents were asked about eleven policy areas: the environment, aid to countries of the former Soviet Union, Social Security, welfare programs, AIDs research, food stamps, public schools, child care, crime, health care, and defense spending. The earlier surveys include some of these spending items, as well as other items that were relevant to a particular year.

Support for Federal Spending: 1984 to 1994

Turning first to general attitudes about government spending, the top panel of Table 9.1 indicates that the public has become a little more likely to support lower levels of spending and fewer services and a little less likely to support higher levels of spending and more services. The proportion of people in the middle of the spending road remained fairly constant over the decade.

Evidence on opinions about spending for particular policy areas appears in the lower panel of Table 9.1. Here we get a rough sense of public priorities, keeping in mind, of course, that the priorities are constrained by the items that respondents were asked to consider. As indicated by the percentage of respondents who thought spending should be increased, funding public schools and dealing with crime have been high priorities across the decade. These priorities are joined by majority support for increased spending on health care, child care, and Social Security in 1994. Majority, or near majority, support for increased spending on Social Security and child care also appears in other election years when the policy area was mentioned.

Although public enthusiasm for increased spending on Social Security has been strong throughout the decade, it has tended to

Table 9.1
Support for Federal Spending, 1984–94

General Attitudes toward Services and Spending:

	1994	1992	1988	1984
(1) Reduce	11	6	6	7
(2)	13	10	10	11
(3)	19	16	16	16
(4)	28	31	29	31
(5)	17	19	18	17
(6)	7	9	12	9
(7) Increase	6	9	9	9
Mean	3.7	4.1	4.1	4.0
N	1567	2018	1615	1866

Attitudes toward Spending for Specific Programs:

	1994			1992			1988			1984		
	more	same	less	more	same	less	more	same	less	more	same	less
Soc. Sec.	52	44	5	49	47	4	59	38	3	52	44	4
Pub. schools	68	25	7	66	30	4	65	30	4	54	40	6
Environment	40	49	11	61	34	4	64	34	3	36	55	8
Food stamps	10	48	43	18	53	30	22	46	32	21	46	33
AIDs	50	36	14	62	30	8	74	20	6			

continued on next page

Table 9.1 (continued)

Attitudes toward Spending for Specific Programs:

	1994			1992			1988			1984		
	more	same	less	more	same	less	more	same	less	more	same	less
Child care	56	34	10	50	40	10	58	32	10	54	42	5
Crime	75	20	5	70	26	3						
Welfare	13	33	54	17	40	42						
Foreign aid*	7	37	56	16	41	43						
Defense	23	48	30							28	47	25
Health care	63	27	9									
Blacks				25	50	24	24	53	23	20	58	21
Unemploy.*				40	48	13	32	54	15	54	32	14
Science*				42	45	13	30	48	21	38	50	11
College stud.				60	32	8	46	43	11			
Homeless				73	21	6	67	28	5			
Big cities				20	50	30						
Poor people				55	38	7						
Drug war							76	20	5			
Contras							12	28	60			
Star Wars							18	34	49			
Elder care							77	22	1			
Medicare										50	45	5
Mean	+.20			+.30			+.32			+.27		
Range of N	1726–1756			2367–2443			1831–1999			1809–1892		

Note: Main entries are percentages of respondents who provided a particular response. Percentages do not always total to 100% due to rounding. The means in the top panel are based on a scale where 1=reduce, 7=increase. Calculation of the means in the bottom panel is described in the text. Programs marked with an asterisk were described in slightly different terms in different years.

lag behind support for increased spending on public schools. In fact, while willingness to spend for Social Security has remained fairly stable, the zeal to fund public schools has grown. Because these questions do not ask respondents to order their preferences, it would be inappropriate to conclude that the public prefers to spend federal funds on school-age children rather than on the elderly. Indeed, two items presented early in the decade do indicate substantial public support for spending on care for the elderly: in 1984 a majority of respondents said that spending for Medicare should be increased; in 1988, 77% of the respondents—more than for any other policy area—wanted to increase spending to care for the elderly. Unfortunately, there are no comparable items from the more recent surveys.[6]

Public restraint in certain policy areas balances the generosity in others. Although respondents usually preferred to maintain current levels of funding rather than decrease them, spending on social assistance programs, defense, and aid to other countries have not been popular during the past decade. Antipathy toward spending in these areas was especially pronounced in 1994. Clear majorities of respondents said they would decrease spending on aid to countries of the former Soviet Union (56%) and welfare (54%), and substantial proportions said they would decrease spending on food stamps (43%) and defense (30%). These patterns are consistent with other evidence that citizens are less likely to support public spending for programs that benefit only a few people, which offer intangible benefits, or that assist people who are perceived as undeserving of the help (Cook and Barrett, 1992; Sanders, 1988; Sears and Citrin, 1982).

Apart from the programs just described, the evidence on public willingness to spend in particular policy areas indicates, as others have noted (Jacoby, 1994, 1995; Sanders, 1988), that frugal attitudes about government expenditures in general do not automatically translate into program-specific thriftiness. If, however, we consider the public's propensity to spend across policy areas, the data do show increasing restraint. The individual spending items were recoded to give each "decrease" response a "−1," each "increase" response a "+1," and each "keep about the same" response a "0." Summing all the spending items in a given year and dividing the sum by the total number of items yields an index with a potential range from "−1" to "+1." The mean scores are shown at the bottom of Table 9.1. They reveal that in the aggregate the public has been more willing to increase spending than to keep it at current levels or decrease it, but this willingness to spend has diminished over the decade.

Age Differences in Support for Federal Spending: 1984 to 1994

Spending Opinion in Four Policy Areas

Four of the spending items—Social Security, public schools, the environment, and food stamps—appear in all four surveys. The first three items are key policy areas in the intergenerational equity discussion. A standard argument forwarded by champions of intergenerational equity is that money spent on retirees is money taken away from programs, such as public education, which benefit the young. Environmental issues also occasionally enter this debate, as proponents of intergenerational equity complain about the shortsightedness and wastefulness of older generations. If there is generational conflict over spending priorities, we should find that the elderly tend to support expenditures on Social Security but not on public schools or the environment, and that younger people tend to do the opposite.[7] In contrast to the other three policy areas, the food stamp program offers social assistance. Helping people in need, perhaps temporarily, and without regard to age, food stamps have nothing to do with intergenerational equity. We should not expect opinions about government spending in this area to vary by age.

The evidence in Table 9.2 confirms some of these predictions. Over the past decade, there have been no significant age differences in support for spending on food stamps. Each year roughly half of each age group has said that spending should be kept about the same. The changes appear in the proportions who prefer more or less spending. By 1994 only about 10% of each age group thought spending on food stamps should increase, compared to twice that level of support in 1984. These changes are fairly uniform across age groups and suggest that the general public has become considerably less enthusiastic about social assistance welfare programs.

Contradicting the generational conflict hypothesis, there have been no significant age differences in the public's willingness to spend on Social Security. Very few people of any age think less money should be spent; the others divide their opinions between keeping expenditures at the same level or increasing them, with some tendency to favor increases. This evidence is entirely consistent with two decades of data on attitudes toward policies and programs that help the elderly (*The Public Perspective*, 1995).

Table 9.2
Age Differences in Support for Federal Spending, 1984-94

	18-34			35-49			50-64			65+		
	more	same	less	more	same	less	more	same	less	more	same	less
Social Security												
1994	55	38	7	49	45	6	54	43	4	49	50	1
1992	49	46	5	49	45	6	52	44	4	44	55	1
1988	61	35	4	63	34	3	57	41	2	52	47	1
1984	54	41	5	56	39	5	49	49	2	45	54	1
Public Schools												
1994*	80	14	6	72	21	7	60	34	6	52	40	8
1992*	75	22	3	66	30	4	57	37	7	55	40	4
1988*	75	23	2	69	28	4	55	38	6	53	41	6
1984*	64	31	4	53	41	6	46	48	7	43	50	7
Environment												
1994*	49	41	10	42	48	10	34	53	14	29	60	11
1992*	67	30	3	61	34	5	55	39	6	57	40	3
1988*	67	30	3	66	32	2	59	38	2	57	39	4
1984*	40	53	7	34	57	9	35	55	10	34	58	8
Food Stamps												
1994	10	47	43	11	46	43	11	47	42	7	51	42
1992	18	51	31	20	51	30	16	56	28	16	56	29
1988	23	46	31	22	41	37	23	48	29	20	51	28
1984	22	40	38	20	48	32	21	52	28	23	50	27

Note: Entries are percentages of respondents who provided a particular response. Percentages do not always total to 100% due to rounding. Asterisks indicate significant age differences in support for spending at p < .05. The number in each age group, from youngest to oldest, is as follows:

1994: 552, 562, 315, 366
1992: 827, 739, 438, 482
1988: 681, 601, 386, 365
1984: 844, 574, 412, 402

Age differences that confirm the generational conflict hypothesis do, however, appear for opinions about spending on public education and the environment. Younger respondents are more likely to favor increasing the amount of funds that go to each of these policy areas; older respondents generally prefer to keep spending at the same level. With respect to the aggregate dynamics of opinions about spending in these two areas, one interesting difference emerges: over the course of the decade older respondents became more willing to increase spending on public schools. Their generosity did not grow any faster than that of the other age groups, but the increase in support that appeared in 1988 has been sustained through the most recent survey.[8] This pattern of relatively lower, but rising, support among the elderly for education spending is consistent with findings from other research (Ponza, et al., 1988).

Determinants of Support for Federal Spending in 1994

The evidence thus far suggests that older Americans are fiscally more conservative than younger citizens, as shown by their opinions about spending in specific policy areas. General attitudes toward government spending follow the same pattern: elderly respondents were significantly more likely to favor lower levels of spending and fewer services during all four years considered here (data not shown). This fiscal conservatism might simply reflect, however, a generally conservative outlook on politics. In 1994, as in the other years under consideration, there was a slight correlation between age and ideological persuasion. Older respondents were more likely to describe themselves as conservative (Pearson's r = −.07, p ≤ .01). Typically, conservatives oppose increases in government spending for the policy areas discussed above; liberals usually support them (Jacoby, 1994). But, the partisan basis of attitudes toward government spending extends beyond ideology to include party. Republicans join conservatives in their opposition to spending increases, while Democrats unite with liberals in their support of them (Eismeier, 1982; Jacoby, 1994; Sanders, 1988). These relationships are not surprising. Nonetheless, they confound the link between age and spending opinion: when older respondents described their party affiliations, they were somewhat more likely than younger respondents to say that they identified as Democrats (Pearson's r = .06, p ≤ .01).

Although the correlations between age and ideology, on the one hand, and age and party, on the other hand, are not strong, they do suggest that the effect of age on attitudes toward government spending may be less straightforward than the generational conflict hypothesis implies. Instead, partisan orientations may affect these attitudes more consistently than age does. What is not clear is whether ideology or party looms larger in determining support for spending in the policy areas we have considered here. If people do not always hold opinions consistent with their age-group interests, are their views more likely to follow their ideological persuasion or their party affiliation? Understanding the role of ideology and party in shaping attitudes toward government spending can provide insight into how citizens of different ages are likely to react to the contemporary partisan debates surrounding budgetary politics.

In addition, there are personal circumstances that may shape an individual's attitudes toward government spending. Respondents with children, for example, might be more likely to support spending on public schools. Respondents who are employed or who have steady incomes might be less sympathetic to the needs of the poor. To the extent that such personal circumstances vary by age, they confound our ability to discern age-specific opinions about public spending in different policy areas. Thus, to evaluate the generational conflict hypothesis we need to look beyond the relationship between age and opinion to consider the effects of partisan and personal factors. Guided by the findings of previous research, the following analysis attempts to take these additional factors into account.

Previous research has shown that attitudes toward government spending are shaped by symbolic political orientations, self-interest, and evaluations of the nation's economy. The premise of the symbolic politics hypothesis is that people acquire stable affective orientations during preadult socialization. These orientations are formed without regard to their future costs or benefits in any particular policy realm and typically include party affiliation, ideological persuasion, group stereotypes, and attitudes toward government (Sears, Hensler, and Speer, 1979; Sears et al., 1980). The perspective is a convenient, recognized way to differentiate a set of influences on opinion from the factors that represent self-interest or personal circumstances. Four symbolic politics variables that have figured in other research on spending attitudes (Jacoby, 1994) are employed: party identification, ideological identification, attitudes about government waste, and symbolic racism.[9] The findings from this research indicate that we should expect less generous opinions about spending among Republicans, conservatives, people who think the government is wasteful, and racists.[10]

Public discussions of Americans' attitudes toward government spending strongly imply that when program cuts hit close to home, people drop all pretenses to thrift. The notion that citizens act on the basis of self-interest has powerfully influenced how elected officials evaluate the likely public response to various policy initiatives (Arnold, 1990). Indeed, what could make more sense than the assertion that people support policies that further their interests and oppose policies that undermine them? Despite the strong intuitive appeal of the self-interest hypothesis, evidence in its favor is mixed. Analyses of attitudes toward public spending have shown that self-interest does shape some spending preferences (Jacoby, 1995; Sanders, 1988), but in other policy areas the effects of self-interest are negligible (Kinder and Sears, 1985).

The most direct example of self-interest with respect to public spending is the receipt of benefits from a government program. The NES surveys sometimes include such variables, but they were not part of the 1994 study.[11] Instead, nine demographic variables are used as proxies for self-interest: age, race, gender, family income, the employment status of the respondent, the highest level of education the respondent has completed, home ownership, the number of children under the age of 18 the respondent has, and the size of the community in which the respondent lived at the time of the interview.[12] Previous research has shown that several of these variables affect general attitudes about government spending (Eismeier, 1982; Jacoby, 1995; Sanders, 1988). Greater support for spending tends to come from racial minorities, women, the unemployed, and people with lower incomes or less education. I expect to find the same here. In addition, I expect certain variables to have program-specific effects. Having children under the age of 18 could increase support for spending on public schools. The size of the community where one resides could influence opinions about spending on the environment; living in a rural area or an urban area may increase awareness of environmental problems and the willingness to pay for solving them. Home ownership imparts a sense of financial security, as well as a sensitivity to tax levels, which could diminish enthusiasm for government spending. Finally, the previous analysis suggests that age will have a negative impact on support for spending in the areas of public education and the environment.

The analysis includes one other variable known to affect general attitudes toward government spending: evaluations of past and future national economic conditions.[13] If we consider that partisan rhetoric connects many economic problems with the federal deficit and excessive government spending, it should not be surprising to find that people who have a pessimistic outlook on the national economy also favor limiting public expenditures (Jacoby, 1995). The same findings are expected here.

Five spending variables provide the dependent measures. One represents general attitudes toward government spending; the other four represent opinions about spending in the policy areas discussed in the previous section: Social Security, public schools, the environment, and food stamps.

Table 9.3 displays the results of the analysis.[14] Turning first to evidence for the symbolic politics hypothesis, we see that two symbolic orientations, party identification and ideological identification, have significant and sizable effects on all five spending variables. As expected, Democrats and liberals generally favor higher levels of government spending and are willing to spend more in each of the four specific policy areas; Republicans and conservatives, not surprisingly, express the opposite attitude toward spending. The impact of the other symbolic orientations is mixed. Although many respondents in the 1994 survey held a dim view of the efficiency of the federal government (71% believed the government wastes tax money), their cynicism fails here to color their attitude toward public spending. Symbolic racism has more pervasive effects: as predicted, racists are less likely to support government spending in general and less likely to endorse spending for food stamps. They are also less willing to spend for the environment, though the reasons for this are not obvious.

The demographic variables that represent self-interest have uneven effects. When they are significant, their effects are generally in the predicted direction. Consider age, the variable of primary interest to this study. The results indicate that, once political orientations and personal considerations have been taken into account, age plays no role in shaping general attitudes toward public spending, nor does it affect opinions about spending for food stamps or Social Security. Clearly, opinions toward spending on the Social Security program have yet to divide the general public in the manner predicted by the intergenerational equity debate. Age does, however, affect views about government funding for public schools and the environment. The older the individual, the less inclined he or she is to support spending in these two policy areas.

To determine whether age has the same effect on opinions about funding other programs whose benefits tend to favor younger citizens, two additional equations based on data from the 1994 NES

Table 9.3
Determinants of Support for Federal Spending, 1994

	Government Spending	Spending for Social Security	Spending for Public Schools	Spending for Environment	Spending for Food Stamps
Party ID (1–7)	.114* (.151)	.015* (.055)	.028* (.100)	.025* (.079)	.035* (.116)
Ideological ID (1–7)	.304* (.243)	.049* (.103)	.100* (.203)	.112* (.211)	.038* (.073)
Wastes taxes (1–3)	-.096 (-.029)	-.018 (-.015)	-.018 (-.014)	-.036 (-.027)	-.045 (-.035)
Racism (1–5)	-.200* (-.115)	.013 (.020)	-.022 (-.034)	-.052* (-.073)	-.109* (-.155)
Age in years (18–91)	-.004 (-.045)	.000 (.012)	-.006* (-.163)	-.004* (-.100)	-.000 (-.012)
Racial minority (1/0)	.055 (.011)	.171* (.097)	.111* (.061)	-.115* (-.059)	.157* (.083)
Female (1/0)	.321* (.100)	.148* (.125)	.126* (.103)	-.004 (-.003)	.001 (.001)
Family income (1–24)	-.021* (-.077)	-.004 (-.038)	.005 (.054)	.002 (.016)	-.017* (-.164)
R employed (1/0)	.139 (.041)	.090* (.072)	.029 (.022)	.010 (.007)	-.088* (-.065)
R's education (1–7)	-.122* (-.122)	-.099* (-.271)	-.039* (-.103)	-.012 (-.029)	-.018* (-.047)
Own home (1/0)	-.034 (-.010)	-.017 (-.014)	-.018 (-.014)	-.077* (-.055)	-.011 (-.008)

	Government Spending	Spending for Social Security	Spending for Public Schools	Spending for Environment	Spending for Food Stamps
Number of kids	.066*	.016	-.003	.008	.018
(0–7)	(.051)	(.033)	(-.006)	(.015)	(.034)
Community size	.020	.004	.006	.006	.010*
(0–8)	(.034)	(.019)	(.029)	(.024)	(.042)
Nat'l economy	-.004	.032*	-.036*	-.021	.001
(1–5)	(-.002)	(.051)	(-.054)	(-.029)	(.001)
Intercept	2.54	1.47	1.48	1.04	0.58
Adjusted R²	.226	.147	.142	.103	.161
N	1297	1435	1440	1442	1427

Note: Main entries are unstandardized OLS coefficients. Entries in parentheses are standardized coefficients. Asterisks denote coefficients significant at p < .05, one-tailed test. The government spending variable ranges from 1 (fewer services/reduce spending) to 7 (more services/increase spending). The other spending variables are coded 0=decrease spending, 1=keep spending the same, 2=increase spending. Dummy independent variables are indicated by (1/0) coding. Ranges for the remaining independent variables are indicated in parentheses below each variable. The extreme values of these ranges are coded as follows: party ID (1=strong Republican, 7=strong Democrat), ideological ID (1=extreme conservative, 7=extreme liberal), government wastes taxes (1=not very much, 3=a lot), symbolic racism (1=low, 5=high), family income (1=less than $3,000, 24=$105,000 and over), respondent's education (1=eighth grade or less, 7=completed advanced degree), community size (0=rural, 8=central city), past and future national economic conditions (1=optimistic perceptions, 5=pessimistic perceptions).

survey were estimated, one for opinions about funding child care and one for opinions about funding AIDs research. Age has a significant (p < .05, one-tailed test) negative effect on both opinions (child care: b = −.006, Beta = −.142; AIDs research: b = −.006, Beta = −.150).

This reluctance of the elderly to spend on programs that would benefit future generations is precisely the selfishness about which proponents of the intergenerational equity issue complain. The concern is that older Americans constitute an increasingly large bloc of active voters who might be able to persuade policymakers to act in accord with the interests of seniors, possibly at the expense of other age groups. At the federal level the elderly could oppose budget reforms they perceive as threatening to the integrity of programs from which they benefit; at the state and local levels they could wield enough clout to defeat referenda on issues that fail to serve their immediate interests (see chapter by MacManus and Tenpas in this volume).

The other demographic variables have sporadic effects on support for spending. Enthusiasm for federal spending is higher among women; urban dwellers; renters; and people with a low family income, less education, and more children. Likewise, members of racial minority groups are more supportive of government spending, unless it is for the environment, a policy area in which minorities are more likely to oppose spending. The effects of employment are also specific to the type of policy area: people who are employed are more likely to support spending on Social Security but less likely to support funding for food stamps.

Finally, evaluations of national economic conditions figure in some spending preferences, although not always in the manner expected. Contrary to findings from previous research, these evaluations fail here to affect general attitudes about government spending. Assessments of the national economy do, however, shape opinions about spending in two specific policy areas. As predicted, pessimistic individuals are less likely to support spending for public schools, but contrary to expectations, they are more likely to support spending for Social Security. Perhaps the link between economic evaluations and spending attitudes is contingent on the benefits individuals anticipate they personally will derive from a particular program. In an economy perceived to be deteriorating, people may be more willing to support government spending on programs from which everyone can reasonably expect tangible benefits, such as Social Security. People may place a much lower priority on funding programs whose benefits are less tangible, or not universally distributed, as in the case of public education.

Support for Federal Spending and
Congressional Vote Choice: 1994

The results of the previous analysis indicate that partisan political identifications are major determinants of public attitudes toward federal spending. Although this is not surprising, it does suggest that the connection between public opinion and public policy turns on the partisan nature of congressional politics. The final analysis of this chapter examines the impact of public opinion about government spending on congressional vote choice. Spending issues were prominent in the 1994 election campaigns of candidates for both the House and the Senate. Candidates from each of the two major parties stressed the need to get the federal budget under control and the need to undertake reforms to entitlement programs, but they also offered party-specific proposals that foreshadowed the partisan differences in approaches to the ongoing budget negotiations. To what extent did voters take these government spending issues into account when casting their ballots in the 1994 elections? Do the issues have effects on vote choice once partisanship has been taken into consideration?

The results in Table 9.4 indicate that certain spending attitudes do indeed have independent effects on voter preference. Three separate sets of models are shown; they differ according to the spending variables included in the vote equations. All variables have been recoded to a zero-one interval to facilitate comparison of the effects. We can begin by noting that party identity and ideological identity always have their expected effects on vote choice, and that these effects are usually the largest ones in the vote models. General attitudes about government spending have a significant effect on voting for House candidates (Model I). Propensity to spend, the index of opinions about spending in eleven policy areas, influences vote choice in House and Senate elections (Model II). In fact, the spending index has an impact on vote choice comparable to the effect of ideological identity. Each version of Model III incorporates a different variable to represent opinion about spending in a specific policy area. Votes for House candidates are affected by opinions about funding for Social Security, public schools, and food stamps; votes for Senate candidates, by opinions about spending on public schools and food stamps. In each case, respondents who favor spending are more likely to support Democrats.

Compared to partisan orientations, policy preferences usually play only a small role in determining vote choices in congressional elections (Jacobson, 1992). The results in Table 9.4 are, thus, not

Table 9.4
Partisanship, Spending Attitudes,
and Congressional Vote Choice, 1994

	House Elections		*Senate Elections*	
Model I:				
Party ID	3.65	(.30)*	3.52	(.33)*
Ideological ID	1.26	(.51)*	3.28	(.60)*
Government spending	.92	(.37)*	−0.14	(.42)
Constant	−2.95	(.24)	−3.37	(.28)
N	862		719	
Model II:				
Party ID	3.76	(.31)*	3.41	(.34)*
Ideological ID	1.08	(.52)*	2.42	(.60)*
Government spending	1.50	(.62)*	2.36	(.74)*
Constant	−3.33	(.35)	−4.31	(.44)
N	828		677	
Model IIIa:				
Party ID	3.75	(.29)*	3.55	(.32)*
Ideological ID	1.42	(.48)*	3.02	(.56)*
Government spending	.70	(.30)*	.04	(.34)
Constant	−3.13	(.30)	−3.31	(.33)
N	912		752	
Model IIIb:				
Party ID	3.86	(.29)*	3.46	(.31)*
Ideological ID	1.29	(.49)*	2.88	(.56)*
Government spending	.58	(.30)*	.76	(.35)*
Constant	−3.10	(.30)	−3.81	(.36)
N	925		762	
Model IIIc:				
Party ID	3.86	(.29)*	3.47	(.31)*
Ideological ID	1.39	(.49)*	2.99	(.56)*
Government spending	.09	(.27)*	.42	(.31)
Constant	−2.75	(.25)	−3.50	(.30)
N	926		763	
Model IIId:				
Party ID	3.90	(.30)*	3.49	(.32)*
Ideological ID	1.12	(.49)*	2.92	(.57)*
Government spending	.67	(.29)*	1.00	(.33)*
Constant	−2.82	(.22)	−3.51	(.28)
N	909		748	

Note: Entries are unstandardized logit coefficients. Entries in parentheses are the standard errors. Asterisks denote coefficients significant at p < .05, one-tailed test. Vote choice is coded 0 for Republican candidates, 1 for Democratic candidates. All independent variables have been recoded to range from 0 (strong Republican, extreme conservative, decrease spending) to 1 (strong Democrat, extreme liberal, increase spending).

exceptional. Policy opinion could, however, play a larger role for certain constituents, especially those for whom a specific program is personally important. To determine whether the effects of spending opinions vary among different constituents, some of the models were respecified to incorporate views about spending on particular programs. This procedure was carried out for each version of Model III in which the main effect of the opinion variable was significant, as shown in Table 9.4. Each revised model includes an interactive term that combines spending opinion with a personal characteristic relevant to the opinion. For the respecified Social Security model (IIIa), the relevant personal characteristic is age; for the public schools model (IIIb), it is age or, in a second respecification of the model, the number of children a respondent has; for the food stamps model (IIId), it is family income. Thus, each fully specified model has four independent variables: party identification, ideological identification, opinion about spending for a particular program, and the interactive term.

The results (not shown) of estimating these revised models offer little support for the hypothesis that opinion about spending for a specific program is more likely to affect the candidate preference of voters for whom the program is personally important. The notable exception is the significant interactive effect of age and opinion about spending on Social Security: older respondents who favor increased spending on Social Security were more likely to vote for Democratic House candidates in 1994 (b = .84, s.e. = .49). Once the interactive term is in the House election model, the main effect of opinion about Social Security spending is rendered nonsignificant (b = .37, s.e. = .35). The only other interactive term with a significant effect is one that combines opinion about public school funding with the number of children a respondent has. It has a significant, but unexpected, effect on voting for House candidates: people with more children and favorable attitudes toward spending on public schools were more likely to vote for Republicans (b = −1.51, s.e. = .62).

These results suggest that the issues central to the intergenerational equity debate play a constrained role in determining vote choice in congressional elections. Opinions about funding Social Security and public schools do figure in voting decisions, and age does intensify the impact of opinion favoring Social Security expenditures, at least for voters in House elections. But, contrary to the generational conflict hypothesis, constituencies defined by age fail here to base their votes on a desire to deny others the benefits of certain programs. The elderly may vote to support a program from which they directly benefit, but they do not seem to be voting in protest of expenditures that benefit future generations.

Conclusion

The analyses in this chapter provide answers to three sets of questions. First, data on general attitudes toward government spending indicate that the public has adopted a slightly more frugal perspective over the decade from 1984 to 1994. Diminished support for spending in general, though, does not always characterize opinions about funding specific programs. Enthusiasm for funding public schools and Social Security, in particular, has remained high.

Second, data on age group differences in spending preferences yield mixed evidence regarding intergenerational conflict over funding priorities. All age groups show similar degrees of support for federal spending on Social Security. The differences emerge for opinions about spending in policy areas whose benefits most directly apply to younger Americans. Specifically, the elderly are less willing than younger citizens to spend for public schools, the environment, child care, and AIDs research; and this age difference in opinion emerges even in multivariate analyses that control for the effects of partisan orientations and personal circumstances.

Third, analyses of voter behavior in the 1994 congressional election confirm that attitudes toward federal spending influence vote choice: fiscal conservatives tend to support Republican candidates, while fiscal liberals are inclined to endorse Democrats. This pattern pertains to general attitudes about government spending as well as specific opinions about spending in policy areas central to the intergenerational equity debate. The effects of spending preferences rarely equal those of party identity or ideological identity, but their influence is consistent enough to suggest that public attitudes toward federal spending are likely to affect the selection of the representatives and senators who will be making future budget decisions. Although the effects of specific opinions tend not to vary across different types of constituents, one notable exception is provided by opinion about spending on Social Security: the older the voter, the larger the impact of this opinion on voting for House candidates.

Proponents of intergenerational equity have for over a decade framed their policy discussions in a manner that highlights the

competing interests of older and younger citizens. Thus far, the
message has failed to undermine public support, in any age group,
for policies that benefit the elderly. But, the evidence presented
here shows that older Americans are not always willing to show
reciprocal support for policies that benefit young people or future
generations. The fiscal conservatism of the elderly is not a recent
development, and to be fair, it extends to a reluctance, relative to
other age groups, to seek increased spending even in policy areas
from which the elderly themselves directly benefit. Of course, we
could also interpret the pattern of opinion toward spending on
Social Security as evidence that senior citizens would resist any
cuts to this program: many think spending should stay at the level
where it has been. These views, coupled with the tendency to turn
out in large numbers at election time (71% of the respondents aged
65 or older voted in the 1994 elections, while only 41% of the
respondents under age 35 did so), have until recently made representatives and senators from both parties unwilling to advocate
fundamental changes to programs that benefit the elderly. The
common presumption is that the large bloc of elderly voters intimi-
dates legislators who might otherwise consider scaling back programs that benefit older Americans. Although not definitive, the
evidence just described indicates that House members do have cause
for concern about the response of older voters to proposals that
threaten Social Security.

The problem is that entitlements for the elderly constitute a
large and growing portion of federal expenditures. One point the
new Republican majority made explicit at the beginning of the
104th Congress is that bringing the federal budget under control
requires legislators to confront many difficult choices, some of which
may alienate constituents whose support they need for reelection.
Recent surveys and focus group discussions suggest, however, that
citizens of all ages are beginning to appreciate the magnitude of
the federal deficit and the need to sacrifice some spending in specific
programs, even ones that have long been "off the table." At the
same time, voters have made clear that they do have preferences,
and not entirely selfish ones, among the possible strategies for
achieving a balanced budget.

The public's spending preferences may influence congressional
decision-making in the short-run, but in the long-run the preferences themselves may be shaped by the character of the policy-
making process. Apart from the details of any particular budget,
the magnitude of the changes legislators have recently proposed

guarantees that the concerns outlined here will continue to shape budget negotiations for several years. Legislators should think of these ongoing deliberations as the beginning of a constructive dialogue about public policy. Although they are accustomed to bargaining with each other in the chambers of Congress, legislators need to consider the impact of their discourse on the public. They have always been mindful of the electoral consequences of their policy choices, but how these choices are presented to the public is also important. In debating their spending priorities, representatives have opportunities to frame policy choices in ways that are either instructive, and likely to foster support and cooperation among diverse constituencies, or divisive, and likely to promote opposition and conflict between competing groups.

Notes

1. AGE directors and staff members published articles in *Atlantic Monthly, Fortune, Newsday, The New York Times, USA Today, The Wall Street Journal*, and the *Washington Post*. The intergenerational equity message also got extensive coverage in a series of articles published by *The New Republic* in 1987.

2. Samuel Preston was perhaps the most influential of these scholars. In his 1984 presidential address to the Population Society of America he established the parameters of the intergenerational equity debate in academic circles by arguing that there is direct competition between the old and the young for society's resources (Preston, 1984).

3. A few legislators from both sides of the aisle have, nonetheless, challenged the "sacred" status of old-age entitlement programs. During the 1995 budget negotiations House Republicans recommended a reduction in the annual cost-of-living adjustment for Social Security and other government benefits, to begin in 1999. They based their proposal on the claim that the price index overstates inflation (Pear, 1995a). At the same time Senator Moynihan (D-NY) offered a similar proposal as an alternative to cutting Medicare and Medicaid (Pear, 1995b). The Republican recommendation was essentially the same plan that Dan Rostenkowski (D-IL), chair of the House Ways and Means Committee, had proposed a year earlier, except that the reduction Rostenkowski suggested would have gone into effect in January 1995. He also proposed to increase the retirement age, trim Social Security benefits for new retirees, and raise payroll taxes in the twenty-first century (Pear, 1994). Reevaluation of old-age entitlement programs has not been limited to Congress. In 1994 President Clinton recognized the need to assess the viability of these programs by forming

the Bipartisan Commission on Entitlement and Tax Reform, a thirty-two-member panel cochaired by Sens. Bob Kerrey (D-NE) and John C. Danforth (R-MO). A few months after the commission made its recommendations, Kerrey and Senator Alan Simpson (R-WY) introduced bipartisan legislation to revamp the Social Security system (*Congressional Record—Senate*, 1995).

4. Codebooks published by the Inter-University Consortium for Political and Social Research describe the sampling procedure and study design. The ICPSR bears no responsibility for the analyses or interpretations presented here.

5. The exact question wording is "Some people think the government should provide fewer services, even in areas such as health and education in order to reduce spending. Suppose these people are at one end of the scale at point 1. Other people feel it is important for the government to provide many more services even if it means an increase in spending. Suppose these people are at the other end, at point 7. And of course, some other people have opinions somewhere in between at points 2, 3, 4, 5, or 6. Where would you place yourself on this scale, or haven't you thought much about this?"

6. The 1992 NES survey includes a separate question about expanding Medicare to pay for nursing home care and long hospital stays for the elderly. Eighty-five percent of the respondents favored or strongly favored doing so; 11 percent opposed or strongly opposed doing so.

7. In light of the overwhelming evidence from previous research that support for Social Security is high among all age groups, we probably should not harbor strong expectations that younger respondents will appear any less supportive in the data reported here. Conflicting priorities may be more apparent in opinions about funding for public schools or the environment. In fact, fear that the elderly are hostile toward government spending in these areas spawned the "gray peril" hypothesis. This hypothesis has found limited support in a series of studies based on aggregate and individual-level data collected throughout Florida (Button, 1992; Button and Rosenbaum, 1990). But, portions of this evidence also indicate that the elderly do not always oppose policies favorable to the interests of other age groups (Rosenbaum and Button, 1989), and that sometimes they strongly support them (Button and Rosenbaum, 1989). Pertinent to the generational conflict hypothesis, Rosenbaum and Button (1993) did, however, find that younger residents of Florida think the priorities of the elderly in their communities are selfish and impose unfair burdens on local government.

8. Other items from the 1994 survey provide further insight into generational differences in attitudes toward spending for particular programs. Older respondents were significantly less willing to fund child care

and AIDs research and significantly more willing to support spending for defense and foreign aid. No significant age group differences appear for opinions about spending on welfare, crime, and health care.

9. Party identification is the standard seven-point NES measure, coded so that low values indicate Republican identity and high values indicate Democratic identity. Ideological identification is another standard seven-point NES measure, with low values representing conservatives and high values representing liberals. Attitudes about government waste are measured by a question that asks respondents whether they think "people in government waste a lot of the money we pay in taxes, waste some of it, or don't waste very much of it." Symbolic racism is a four-item scale based on questions about the status of blacks in American society. The series of questions is introduced with the following statement: "In past studies we have asked people why they think white people seem to get more of the good things in life in America—such as better jobs and more money—than black people do. These are some of the reasons given by both blacks and whites." Respondents are asked whether they agree strongly, agree some-what, neither agree nor disagree, disagree somewhat, or disagree strongly. The specific statements are: "Over the past few years, blacks have gotten less than they deserve." "Irish, Italians, Jewish and many other minorities overcame prejudice and worked their way up. Blacks should do the same without any special favors." "It's really a matter of some people not trying hard enough; if blacks would only try harder they could be just as well off as whites." "Generations of slavery and discrimination have created conditions that make it difficult for blacks to work their way out of the lower class." These questions were posed to respondents of all races. The first and fourth items were reflected in constructing the symbolic racism scale (Cronbach's alpha = .71).

10. Racists' opposition to government spending on social assistance programs is based on the perception that black people do not deserve the help such programs provide (Sniderman and Piazza, 1993).

11. Previous research indicates these variables have limited effects on support for public spending (see Sanders, 1988; Jacoby, 1995; and Rhodebeck, 1993).

12. Race, gender, employment status, and home ownership are dummy variables coded "1" for respondents who are racial minorities, women, working 20 or more hours a week, and owning a home. Age is coded in years from 18 to 91; family income, in 24 categories that range from $2,999 or less to $105,000 or more; education, in seven categories that range from eighth grade education or less to completion of an advanced degree; number of children, none to seven; size of community, in nine categories that range from rural to central city.

13. This variable is the sum of two items. One asked respondents whether they thought the economy in the country as a whole had gotten

better, stayed about the same, or gotten worse over the past year. The other asked if they expected the economy to get better, stay the same, or get worse. The summated index ranges from "much better" to "much worse."

14. The use of OLS regression is really only appropriate for the equation in which "government spending" is the dependent variable. The other spending variables are three category ordinal scales. Multinomial logit or polychotomous probit are the appropriate models for estimating the equations in which these variables appear. I report the results of OLS estimation to facilitate comparison across the five equations. The results of the polychotomous probit estimations do not differ substantively from the OLS estimations.

References

Arnold, R. Douglas. (1990). *The Logic of Congressional Action*. New Haven: Yale University Press.

Berke, Richard L. (1995). Poll finds public doubts key parts of G.O.P.'s agenda. *New York Times*, 28 February, p. A–1.

Broder, David. (1995). Changes ahead for Medicare. *San Francisco Examiner*, 29 July, p. A–15.

Butterworth, Nicholas. (1993). Generation X marks the spot. *New York Newsday*, 14 July, part 2.

Button, James W. (1992). A sign of generational conflict: The impact of Florida's aging voters on local school and tax referenda. *Social Science Quarterly*, 73, 786–97.

———, and Rosenbaum, Walter A. (1989). Seeing gray: School bond issues and the aging in Florida. *Research on Aging*, 11, 158–73.

———. (1990). Gray power, gray peril, or gray myth?: The political impact of the aging in local Sunbelt politics. *Social Science Quarterly*, 71, 25–38.

Congressional Record—House. Thursday, 25 May 1995, 141st *Congressional Record* H 5607, Vol. 141 No. 88, Public Bills and Resolutions.

Congressional Record—Senate. Thursday, 18 May 1995 (Legislative Day of Monday, 15 May 1995), 141st *Congressional Record* S 6912, Vol. 141 No. 83, Introduction of Bills and Joint Resolutions.

Cook, Fay Lomax, and Barrett, Edith J. (1992). *Support for the American Welfare State: The Views of Congress and the Public*. New York: Columbia University Press.

Day, Christine L. (1990). *What Older Americans Think: Interest Groups and Aging Policy.* Princeton: Princeton University Press.

Deets, Horace B. (1994). Anticipating the 1995 WHCoA. *Modern Maturity,* 37, 6–7.

Eismeier, Theodore J. (1982). Public preferences about government spending: Partisan, social, and attitudinal sources of policy differences. *Political Behavior,* 4, 133–45.

Fraley, Colette. (1995). Medicare cuts yet to be fleshed out. *Congressional Quarterly Weekly Reports,* 53, 1900.

Hager, George. (1993). Entitlements: The untouchable may become unavoidable. *Congressional Quarterly Weekly Report,* 51, 22–30.

Jacobson, Gary C. (1992). *The Politics of Congressional Elections. 3d ed.* New York: Harper Collins.

Jacoby, William G. (1994). Public attitudes toward government spending. *American Journal of Political Science,* 38, 336–61.

———. (1995). Issue Framing and Public Opinion on Government Spending. Prepared for presentation at the 1995 Annual Meetings of the Midwest Political Science Association, Chicago.

Kinder, Donald R., and Sears, David O. (1985). Public opinion and political action. In Gardner Lindzey and Eliot Aronson (Eds.), *Handbook of Social Psychology. Vol. 2, Third Edition.* New York: Random.

Kingson, Eric R. (1988). Generational equity: An unexpected opportunity to broaden the politics of aging. *The Gerontologist,* 28, 765–72.

Kolbert, Elizabeth. (1995). Shifting public opinion by a turn of phrase. *New York Times,* 5 June, p. A–1.

Lacayo, Richard. (1993). Remember the deficit? *Time,* 142 (8 November), 39–40.

MacManus, Susan A. (1995). Taxing and spending politics: A generational perspective. *The Journal of Politics,* 57, 607–29.

Pear, Robert. (1994). To shore up Social Security, cuts and tax rises are urged. *New York Times,* 19 April, p. A–12.

———. (1995a). G.O.P. suggests smaller benefit adjustments. *New York Times,* 11 May, p. B–12.

———. (1995b). Senate eyes cuts in Social Security. *The New York Times,* 27 September, p. A–1.

Ponza, Michael, Duncan, Greg J., Corcoran, Mary, and Groskind, Fred. (1988). The guns of autumn? Age differences in support for income transfers to the young and old. *Public Opinion Quarterly,* 52, 441–66.

Preston, Samuel H. (1984). Children and the elderly: Divergent paths for America's dependents. *Demography*, 21, 435–58.

The Public Perspective. (1995). Social Security: American icon. February/ March.

Quadagno, Jill. (1989). Generational equity and the politics of the welfare state. *Politics and Society*, 17, 353–76.

Rhodebeck, Laurie A. (1993). The politics of greed? Political preferences among the elderly. *The Journal of Politics*, 55, 342–64.

Rosenbaum, Walter A., and Button, James W. (1989). Is there a gray peril?: Retirement politics in Florida. *The Gerontologist*, 29, 300–306.

———. (1993). The unquiet future of intergenerational politics. *The Gerontologist*, 33, 481–90.

Rubin, Alissa J. (1995). Medicare: Throwing down the gauntlet. *Congressional Quarterly Weekly Report*, 53, 1304.

Sanders, Arthur. (1988). Rationality, self-interest, and public attitudes on public spending. *Social Science Quarterly*, 69, 311–24.

Sears, David O., and Citrin, Jack. (1982). *Tax Revolt: Something for Nothing in California*. Cambridge: Harvard University Press.

Sears, David O., Hensler, Carl P., and Speer, Leslie K. (1979). Whites' opposition to 'Busing': Self-interest or symbolic politics. *American Political Science Review*, 73, 369–84.

Sears, David O., Lau, Richard R., Tyler, Tom R., and Allen, Jr., Harris M. (1980). Self-interest vs. symbolic politics in policy attitudes and presidential voting. *American Political Science Review*, 74, 670–84.

Sniderman, Paul M., and Piazza, Thomas. (1993). *The Scar of Race*. Cambridge: Harvard University Press.

Social Security Bulletin. (1995). Actuarial status of the Social Security and Medicare programs. 58, 58–64.

Strauss, Melanie, and Dee, Gretchen. (1995). No serious dialogue. *Future Focus*, July, p. 1.

Thau, Rich. (1995). To our members. *Future Focus*, July, p. 1.

Third Millennium Declaration. (1993). New York: Third Millennium.

Toner, Robin. (1995a). G.O.P. feels the heat. The furnace: Medicare. *New York Times*, 5 May, p. A–20.

———. (1995b). Senate approves welfare plan that would end aid guarantee. *New York Times*, 20 September, p. A–1.

Part III

THE FAMILY, ETHNICITY, AND OLDER WOMEN:
AGING POLICY DILEMMAS

Chapter 10

Changing Family Demographics, Caregiving Demands,
and the Policy Environment

TONYA M. PARROTT

The atmosphere in Washington, D.C., today suggests that more
emphasis will be placed on the obligation of the family to take responsibility for the needs of their own aging family members. The
paradox, however, is that families *already* provide 80% of the informal care received by the elderly (Cantor, 1983; Stone, Cafferata, and
Sangl, 1987). One national study estimated that 4.2 million spouses
and children were caregivers to disabled elders and another 13.5
million individuals had the potential to become caregivers (Stone
and Kemper, 1989). The crux of this contradictory situation is whether
family members can be expected to take on *more* care of aging relatives at a time when dramatic social and political changes in American society are having a major impact on family life. Many questions
are raised by proposals to scale back federal programs such as Social
Security and Medicare and by the prospects of turning over control
of programs such as Medicaid to the states in the form of block
grants. As the rhetoric for individual and family responsibility gains
more legitimacy as an organizing principle for policy, it is essential
to look at what is already occurring in families and what will likely
occur in the future. This chapter first reviews the policy assumptions
made about aging families, and then outlines major research findings
in the areas of family demography, intergenerational support, and
heterogeneity across families. This is followed by a discussion of the
current policy environment in which issues of family responsibility

and caregiving have been raised. Proposals for the future that take into account the policy context are presented last.

Policy Assumptions about Aging Families

Assumptions about family life are routinely made by policy-makers. However, in terms of the policy definitions used, there is no clear agreement on what a "family" really is (Moen and Schorr, 1988; Chalfie, 1995). Some policies that assist families use a definition based on marital relations or lineage while other policies define families based on who provides care and attends to material needs. Each definition is also open to political attack because it denies benefits to some family forms while legitimating others.

Although there is no single, comprehensive aging family policy in the United States, there are numerous examples of policies designed to help families in caregiving situations, and these include the following: the Family and Medical Leave Act; tax breaks and financial compensation to caregivers (Linsk et al., 1992); adult day-care centers (Bradsher, Estes, and Stuart, 1995); state-level filial responsibility laws (Bulcroft, Van Leynseele, and Borgatta, 1989); benefits to grandparents raising grandchildren (Mullen, 1995); and the wide array of supportive services in communities that aim to help families and older individuals maintain care arrangements at home rather than in institutions (Liebig, 1993). Each of these policies have varying definitions of who can use them, how they are financed, who is responsible for paying if the elderly individual cannot, and who is considered eligible for benefit payments as a caregiver. Family form, family income, living arrangements, and level of need all come in to play and are related to larger issues of what a family is and the assumptions made by policymakers about family life and family responsibilities.

Policy Assumptions

Five assumptions that permeate policy proposals for families are particularly relevant to the situation and needs of aging families. First, many policymakers assume family concerns are focused on the child-rearing years, where premarital sex, affordability of college, and keeping children safe and away from drugs are often predominant concerns (Moen and Forest, 1995). Indeed, it could be argued that no comprehensive *aging family* policy exists. Rather, much policy devoted to the needs of the elderly focuses on the *individual older person* rather than on families trying to cope with problems that arise as family members age. Issues that impact the lives of the elderly, including economic well-being and affordability of long-term care, are family concerns because older persons rely on family members for a great deal of informal assistance (Stone, Cafferata, and Sangl, 1987). Help and support that cannot be provided by the family is usually sought from the community. For example, many working families rely on community-based services such as Dial-a-Ride and Meals-on-Wheels programs to help transport seniors to doctor appointments or socialization activities and to take care of their nutritional needs during the workday.

As children age and move out of their parents' homes, family concerns may shift from raising children to the needs of aging parents and grandparents. Indeed, helping parents adjust to the changes of old age can be considered an expected event for aging adult children (Brody, 1990). For example, if a mother is widowed, can no longer take care of her household, has poor eyesight, and the only adult child lives in another state, long-distance arrangements must be made either to get assistance to the parent or to relocate the parent to a retirement home. Alternatively, consideration may be given to moving the mother to the son or daughter's town or into his or her own home. It has even been suggested that decisions made by adult children to accept or not accept job promotion transfers to other geographic locations have been tempered by the real or anticipated care needs of older parents (Scharlach and Boyd, 1989). These are all tough choices that only begin to become important around the time that an individual's child rearing years are ending. Thus, the conclusion that family policy is a life course issue is certainly valid (Moen and Forest, 1995). Moreover, at the same time that parent care may become a growing concern for adult children, the onset of their own health problems may rise to the surface as a developing problem requiring attention.

A second assumption often made by policymakers is that if government assistance were offered to families with aging relatives, then family members would stop providing informal, free care and would instead take advantage of the opportunity to be financially compensated for their services or to purchase formal care. Studies done in several states find that this "substitution effect" anticipated by many politicians is not occurring in programs where compensation has been offered to family caregivers who assist older relatives (Linsk et al., 1992; Seccombe, 1992; Gerald, 1993). In short, formal services are not a substitute for the familiarity of a family member, even though such services may be helpful in cases where a family caregiver works and does not have a flexible schedule or for situations in which a family care organizer lives in a different state from the older family member in need of assistance. Linsk et al. (1992: 31) conclude that, "Policymakers' concern about families abusing a compensation policy appear to be based on fears and attitudes rather than data."

Some policymakers and business owners feel that if a policy were passed that mandated that caregivers who work be given time off to take care of family needs or be given flexible schedules in order to carry out care obligations, then the worker would be less productive, the lost productivity would be an added expense to the business, and that there would be a "woodwork effect" where more workers than estimated would take advantage of the policy (Scharlach and Boyd, 1989; Gerald, 1993). Recent analyses of eldercare programs, however, have found otherwise.

Eldercare refers to specific programs and policies in the workplace that are designed to help employees who are caregivers. Employees who provide care to the elderly put themselves at risk for experiencing job interferences, missed income because of unpaid leave, and foregone opportunities for job promotions; employers have costs due to caregiving that are associated with caregiver absenteeism, hiring replacement workers and training them, and lost productivity due to work-family distractions and conflicts (Gottlieb, Kelloway, and Fraboni, 1994). The establishment of eldercare programs appears to eliminate or diminish these problems. Offering time off, flexible work schedules, financial benefits, and information referral improves the well-being of some employed caregivers (Barr, Johnson, and Warshaw, 1992). As for fears that eldercare programs would be overutilized, participation by employees runs between 4% and 5%; when employees take time off to provide care, four-fifths of them take off five days or less (ibid.).

The Family and Medical Leave Act (FMLA) of 1993 is a policy designed to give workers in businesses with over fifty employees up to twelve weeks unpaid leave a year to, among other things, care for a child, spouse, or parent with a serious health condition. A report on the FMLA to a bipartisan commission charged with monitoring the act concluded that only about 3% of eligible workers took advantage of the policy for *any* of the covered reasons. However, 60% of workers in the United States are not covered by this national policy (U.S. Department of Labor, 1993). Thus, assumptions about substitution and woodwork effects appear unsupported in practice.

A third assumption that predominates in policy arenas is that *families* are responsible for the care of older relatives and thus *government* does not have the primary responsibility of figuring out how to take care of this matter. Thus, there is much resistance to public intervention into what is still perceived as a private problem. This view can be seen in arguments used against state policies that financially compensate family caregivers for their efforts. Some opponents of government involvement in family life have argued that paying family caregivers would change the nature of the relationship from one of affection and intimacy to a contractual relationship that could potentially be corrupted by a desire to be reimbursed for a "caring" act (Doty, 1986).

While there is a strong norm of family responsibility toward elders in the United States, it is not always the case that family members are able to carry out these obligations (Finley, Roberts, and Banahan, 1988). Even if a strong sense of *normative obligation* as well as a strong *desire* to help family members endure, the *ability* to help an older relative either by giving time or financial assistance may not exist (Wolfson, et al., 1993). By assuming that families should care for older relatives, policymakers can absolve themselves of the problems of old age and reduce spending or allocate funding to other sources.

Fourth, it is assumed that somehow families are not doing enough to help older relatives and that they could be doing more if forced to do so. This point is illustrated in the GOP Medicaid Transformation Act proposed during the 104th Congress. While vetoed by President Clinton, this proposal has not disappeared from the political agenda. It would allow states to require that adult children with incomes greater than the state median income have to help pay for the nursing home bills of a parent who is receiving Medicaid funds. This proposal makes the assumption that family members have not done enough to assist their aging parents and that they should be required to do more. What this proposal ignores, but policies of financial compensation to caregivers presume, is that family care is not "costless." Several researchers have estimated the wages foregone by informal family caregivers: an average wage of $6.23 an hour (White-Means and Chollet, 1996); $9.40 to $10.30 per hour (Ernst and Hay, 1994); $29.15 per day (Hu, Huang, and Cartwright, 1986). In light of this foregone financial compensation, assuming—much less mandating—that families should give more assistance to the frail, disabled elderly appears unsupportable as a policy assumption.

In some cases it may be true that if a program is cut families will figure out a way to pick up the slack and survive, but at what cost to family life, individual well-being, and family resources? If an adult child is required to fund the nursing home care of an older parent, savings that were supposed to pay for the college education of children or for the adult child's own retirement years and health care needs are put at risk. Changes in one policy area have ramifications far beyond the individual elderly recipient (Zimmerman, 1988); families are forced to pinch-hit in ways that may be unrealistic because they require too much of a sacrifice from younger generations for older generations in the family. The still unanswerable question for the future is whether or not families can do more than they are already doing and still be prepared for the other contingencies of family life and old age.

A last assumption about caregiving in general, and reflected in public policies that do attempt to address caregiving issues for families, is that there is a single, identifiable caregiver who performs the care responsibilities for an older person. Studies have shown that while there may be a primary caregiver, there are also usually secondary caregivers. Moreover, if there are multiple caregivers, often they perform different tasks, all of which are necessary and needed by the care recipient (Lee, Dwyer, and Coward, 1993). In some families, caregivers are rotated, with an older parent living with one child for four months of the year, another child for four months, and a third child for another four months. Families work out unique caregiving arrangements as best they can given competing demands on time and resources. Indeed, an argument against having a family policy for caregivers is that family members would lose their freedom to arrange these varied caring relationships if a standardized national or state family policy were put in place that stipulated which types of family care were reimbursable and which were not (Seccombe, 1992).

Given the variety of assumptions about aging families, to what extent are these assumptions grounded in evidence and supported by current knowledge about aging, caregiving, and the family? The next sections review the changing demography of family life, implications for intergenerational support, and the heterogeneity of family care needs in today's aging society.

Demographics of Family Life

Although there has been a decline in the number of persons born into each generation in a family during the twentieth Century, there are more people up and down the family lineage living longer and spending a larger proportion of their lives in intergenerational relationships than ever before in American history (Bengtson, Rosenthal, and Burton, 1990). The increased longevity of the older population has opened up the opportunity for parents and their adult children to spend a longer portion of their lives in *adult* relationships rather than in parent-child relationships (Uhlenberg, 1980, 1993). Not only have grandchildren been able to get to know their grandparents, but the increased life span of grandparents has given grandchildren the opportunity to have mature and developed relationships with their grandparents *after* the grandchild reaches adulthood (Hodgson, 1992; Robertson, 1995). Moreover, great-grandchild and great-grandparent relationships have become more common (Ahlburg and De Vita, 1992). The flip side of this increase in the number of generations living at one time is that there are fewer persons within each generation alive and there are more people in the middle-age generation choosing to have fewer children or to remain childless. The consequence is that there will be fewer adult children available to assist aging parents in the future (Myers, 1992). In the Baby Boom generation (those born between 1946 and 1964) for example, nearly 16% of women between the ages of 40 and 44 have not yet had children and are likely to remain childless (Treas, 1995).

Contact across the generations remains high as family members age, contrary to the persistent myth that families have abandoned their elders and neglect them in old age (Shanas, 1979; Bengtson, Rosenthal, and Burton, 1996). Older family members remain integrated in family life and despite the mobility that today's work force requires, elders continue to have frequent contact—either in-person or by telephone and mail—with their adult children. Although it has been suggested that the generations are being separated by geographic mobility, thus threatening the availability of informal social support to older persons, Uhlenberg (1993) argues that there is no empirical evidence to suggest that there is a trend toward extended families being split across state boundaries. In a recent study of intergenerational relationships, the majority of adult children lived within one hour of at least one parent (Lawton, Silverstein, and Bengtson, 1994a).

While many older persons prefer living on their own compared to living with an adult child, and most are able to do so, as women grow older and outlive their husbands, they may eventually have to move in with an adult child or other relative when a need arises. For example, Treas (1995) showed that of women 75 years and older living in the community, 20% were living with a relative other than a spouse in 1994. In contrast, of men aged 75 or older in 1994, 7% lived with a relative other than a spouse. Part of this difference is reflected in the longer life expectancy and higher rates of widowhood for women (see chapter by Steckenrider in this volume).

More middle-aged and older adults, especially older women, are living in nontraditional households. A recent study by Chalfie (1995) of the prevalence of nontraditional living arrangements (e.g., grandparent caregivers, extended families, and partners and room-mates) found that 15% to 17% of all individuals live in these non-traditional households, and more than half of the individuals are female. Twenty-four percent of these nontraditional households are adults 45 and older: 16% are aged 45 to 64 and 8% are 65 and older. Women who were divorced, never married, or widowed were the most likely to live in these nontraditional households.

The family demographic scenario for the Baby Boomers points to some important trends as well (Bouvier and De Vita, 1991; De Vita, 1996): divorce and remarriage rates are higher for this generation than for previous generations, labor force participation rates for women are higher in this generation, and more couples in this group are cohabitating rather than marrying. There has also been a rise in the number of persons choosing to remain single or involved in homosexual relationships. It has been suggested that these changes in marital status will result in an unstable support network in old age. Indeed, as this cohort ages their *access* to family members may be altered by divorce and remarriage as well as by labor force participation (Seccombe, 1992; Lawton, Silverstein, and Bengtson, 1994b). The implications of these changes for intergenerational support are explored next.

Implications of Aging Family Demographics
for Intergenerational Support

Working-age Baby Boomers face many uncertainties as they begin to turn fifty years old, including fewer guarantees of steady employment until the retirement years arrive, wage stagnation and dimmer prospects for increased earnings in the later years of life, job discrimination if they seek employment at older ages, and the likelihood that their savings may not be enough to allow them to retire (Bouvier and De Vita, 1991; De Vita 1996). Indeed, many Baby Boomers may find that they have to continue to work longer than anticipated and for lower wages than expected. Added to these labor market conditions, however, is the knowledge that more and more women are entering the paid labor force and contributing to their own pension plans and family income (Shank, 1988).

There has been a great amount of concern that older working women will be forced to make a choice between their jobs or caring for an older family member at a time in their lives when they may need to earn an income to prepare for their own retirement and old age needs (Brody, 1990; Thomas, 1993; Stephens and Franks, 1995). Recent research indicates, however, that despite the predictions of women being forced to leave the labor market for caregiving responsibilities, the trade-off between employment and family care obligations does not occur for all caregivers.

Studies of employees show that one-fifth to one-third are caregivers for the elderly (Barr, Johnson, and Warshaw, 1992). Thus, not all caregivers are in the paid labor force. However, women who work full-time are more likely to become family caregivers than are their fully employed male counterparts (ibid.). In fact, working women have been found just as likely to take on caregiving responsibilities as nonworking women (Seccombe, 1992; Moen, Robison, and Fields, 1994; Robison, Moen, and Dempster-McClain, 1995). An intriguing explanation for the same life chances of becoming a caregiver for these two sets of women was offered by Robison et al. (1995): working women have developed skills that allow them to juggle roles between family and work life and thus they have the adaptive resources necessary to commit to an additional family obligation.

Notably, working women may be forced to rely on formal services more than nonworking caregiving women because of time constraints that make formal care options desirable. Moreover, the type of employment a caregiver has (blue-collar vs. white-or pink-collar) may allow the caregiver less (in the case of blue-collar) or more (in the case of white- and pink-collar) job flexibility to accommodate caregiving responsibilities (Starrels, et al., 1995). Workplace studies show that between 10% and 20% of employed caregivers report a job exit, early retirement, or time-off without pay due to caregiving responsibilities (Stone, Cafferata, and Sangl, 1987; Scharlach, Lowe, and Schneider, 1991). Kingson and O'Grady-LeShane (1993) estimate that these early exits from the labor force by caregivers result in Social Security monthly benefits that are approximately $127 lower than if the caregiver had remained in the work force.

Other important demographic trends among Baby Boomers also highlight the complex relationship between caregiving arrangements and family structure. For example, with higher rates of divorce among older Baby Boomers, these adult children may be made more vulnerable to economic conditions and thus even less capable of assisting older family members in need. In this case, while the desire to help might exist, the ability to help both emotionally and financially would be greatly reduced (Cicirelli, 1983). Rather, adult children may turn to their aging parents for emotional and financial support. For instance, aging parents often perform an important role in the lives of grandchildren when a divorce among adult children occurs (Robertson, 1995). In one study, divorced daughters with custody of children received more help from their parents than did married daughters (Spitze et al., 1994). If aging parents are facing their own physical frailties and rising health care needs at the same time that their adult children are experiencing divorce, these are competing demands on family resources that can test the buffering qualities of the family social support network. However, Spitze et al. (1994) found that, following a divorce, daughters did not decrease their assistance to parents. If an adult child becomes widowed, his or her time and ability to assist an aging parent may actually increase (Brody et al., 1994). At times, family events can have both negative and positive outcomes; while the loss of a mate can be devastating, the loss can also mean increased attention and exchanges of assistance between parents and adult children. Thus, not all negative life events have negative policy consequences.

An equally complex demographic change within families is the remarriage of an adult child. Indeed, most individuals who divorce are likely to remarry (De Vita, 1996). Remarriages offer blended, step-, and half-family relationships that some researchers suggest may weaken the family support network (Johnson, 1993). Daughters-in-law often provide the informal support needed by aging parents-in-law. If a divorce occurs, the female caregiver may withdraw her support to her ex-parents-in-law. When a divorce occurs, contact is usually maintained with the custodial grandparents, often the maternal grandparents, and thus the noncustodial grandparents lose any hope of this potential caregiving source. This creates a caregiving dilemma for the male ex-spouse and his parents. Add to this configuration the remarriage of the female ex-spouse and it is easy to see how a once stable care arrangement can disappear.

Divorce among aging parents, no longer as uncommon as it once was, is also an area of demographic family change that should be of concern to policymakers (Uhlenberg, Cooney, and Boyd, 1990). Lawton, Silverstein, and Bengtson (1994b), for example, have found that when a divorce occurs among aging parents, adult children often lose contact with the aging father while contact is maintained with the aging mother. Reasons for this vary from gender differences in kin-keeping practices to studies showing that relationships with mothers tend to be closer than those with fathers (Cooney and Uhlenberg, 1990; Bulcroft and Bulcroft, 1991). When a divorce occurs between aging parents, it appears that the elderly father is the most vulnerable to the loss of social support while the elderly mother is more likely to retain her social support network. Moreover, older wives are most likely to be the primary caregivers to their older husbands (for a discussion of gender differences in spousal caregiving see Allen, 1994; also see chapter by Steckenrider in this volume). Thus, following a divorce, the older husband not only has a higher likelihood of losing the support of his children, but also of his primary caregiver—his wife.

Remaining childless (or "child free") is an option with seemingly dramatic implications for caregiving arrangements in later life. Aside from a spouse, the daughter or daughter-in-law usually provides care to the aging family member in long-term care situations (Hooyman, 1992). Sons also provide care, although when there is a daughter nearby it is more often the daughter who takes over the primary responsibility for care arrangements (Matthews, 1992). For couples or older individuals who choose to remain childless and for the aging Baby Boomers who have chosen not to have children, what will happen to their first lines of support in old age? At this point, the evidence suggests that these individuals are more likely to rely on siblings, other kin including nieces and nephews, and neighbors and friends for informal social support (Genevay, 1993). Formal support is also more likely to be used. Again, older women seem to fare better than older men because older women tend to spend their younger lives developing networks of friends and kin whom they can then call upon in old age whereas men are more likely to depend on their wives and do not develop outside networks of potential caregivers. Older men are more at risk in terms of later life caregiving needs compared to older women, but the likelihood of an older man being unmarried in later life and living alone is very low compared to the rates of widowhood and living alone for older women (Treas, 1995). Thus, while older men may seem more vulnerable than older women to these circumstances, they are less likely to end up in these situations.

Baby Boomers will have more siblings available in later life than previous generations have had to rely on, thus the supposed dilemma proposed by childlessness and remaining single may be partially offset by this fact of greater sibling availability (Bedford, 1995). As with other family relationships, however, the availability of a sibling may not translate into actual caregiving between siblings; this may vary based on the quality of the earlier relationship, number of siblings, and whether or not the relationship is full, half, or step in nature (Connidis, 1994).

Among Baby Boomers (as well as among their children) there is a growing trend toward cohabitation and never marrying (Bouvier and De Vita, 1991). This living arrangement has important caregiving implications because it means that the traditional caregiving that occurs between aging couples may or may not be forthcoming in this situation, especially if the cohabitation ceases in later life. Moreover, cohabitation arrangements lack the legal entitlement to benefits associated with marriage such as tax breaks for married couples and the right to survivor's benefits after death (Chalfie, 1995). Two aspects of such living arrangements and marital status choices are overlooked: (1) policymakers may not be recognizing or assessing the availability of nonkin social supports and their meaning to older individuals; and (2) being classified as "nonmarried" might afford older individuals some policy opportunities—namely, they may qualify for social service benefits because they are not married and, as a result, are identified as "at risk" (even if they do have a life partner or roommate). A study of nontraditional living arrangements concluded that in many cases nontraditional households "have an edge over traditional households in qualifying for some public benefits" (ibid.). Thus, from a policy standpoint, it would be wise to account for nonkin supportive relationships and to examine the conditions under which eligibility for caregiving benefits are allocated. For example, is it fair to deny caregiving payments to kin but to give caregiving payments to roommates or partners who are considered nonkin by policy definitions? Such diverse care arrangements are addressed in the next section.

Diversity and Heterogeneity in Caregiving Experiences and Needs

Not only do changing family demographics have caregiving implications, but the diversity and heterogeneity of family caregiving situations must also be considered when talking about policies for aging families. First, mentally and physically handicapped children are living longer lives due to innovations and developments in the health field (Sutton, 1993). Retarded children, for example, are now living into their 50s and older. The aging parents of these adult children cannot rely on their children for social support in old age, and they may still be providing social support to these children as they themselves age and need assistance. Two important policy questions arise in these aging family situations: (1) Who will care for the aging parent? (2) Who will care for the aging child with physical or mental impairments when the parents become too frail to do so? These dilemmas for families and public policy are relatively new and are only beginning to be addressed (Smith et al., 1995). The increased demand on state assistance to the disabled is tested as these adult children live longer at the same time that an older parent's need for long-term formal assistance may emerge. Trade-offs and policy choices between these two generations may be faced as they essentially compete for long-term care resources from the states and federal government. Although the numbers of families in this situation may be small in absolute terms, the cost of such caregiving arrangements and the need to openly discuss such situations cannot be underestimated.

A second trend that is important again applies to family situations where it is the child, rather than the older parent, who initiates the dilemma: as the AIDS epidemic grows and as alcohol and drug dependencies push the limits of family strength, several caregiving dilemmas arise. Similar to the situation with mentally and physically handicapped adult children, it is becoming more common for parents to be asked to care for their sick and dying adult children who have contracted the AIDS virus. The same issues arise here as well regarding who will care for the aging parent and who will care for the dying child if the parent dies first or becomes too ill to care for the adult child. Indeed in 1989 the journal *Generations* devoted an entire issue to the problems raised by AIDS and caregiving. Related to this issue is the situation of grandparents raising grandchildren because either the adult child has contracted AIDS or because the adult child has a drug or alcohol dependency that takes him or her out of the home or that requires the adult child to give up (even if only temporarily) custody of his or her children (Chalfie, 1994). Again, the situation is arising such that aging parents who are facing retirement or who are already retired are being called upon to become caregivers for small children (Jendrek, 1993). Not only is the physical and mental health of the grandparent put at risk, but so are the financial resources of the grandparent, resources that may be very necessary for his or her survival in retirement (Presser, 1989; Minkler, Roe, and Price, 1992). Some public policies are emerging to address the needs of grandparents who have become caregivers, but the benefits available are often limited or are only available to grandparents who are poor or who have sole custody of their grandchildren (Mullen, 1995). For example, in efforts to trim budgets, some states (e.g., New York) are proposing limiting foster care payments and other supportive payments to grandparents.

A third trend of importance to caregiving policy for aging families is the rise in the incidence of dementia, especially Alzheimer's Disease, with advanced age. As more and more older individuals are living into old age, the chance of getting this form of dementia grows and the likelihood of a family member facing care for a demented loved one grows as well (Hodgson and Cutler, 1994). Because the needs of many Alzheimer's patients are custodial and long-term in orientation, rather than acute conditions for which Medicare funds may be used, few services are available to families that are funded through public support programs. While some communities do have social support services for family members caring for demented elders, this set of family caregivers is often at the end of their capability to care for the demented elder by the time they turn to formal care services for assistance (George and Gwyther, 1986; Wright, Clipp, and George, 1993). Thus the limits of family care and family responsibility are being reached in situations where the older family member develops Alzheimer's Disease. It seems unlikely that policymakers could expect families in these situations to do more.

Homosexual relationships among Baby Boomers is a fourth diverse family caregiving situation. Given that all states (and most companies) deny spousal benefits to nonheterosexual partners as well as the congressional and public movement to deny same-sex marriages, how do these family care arrangements manifest themselves in old age and what are the implications for caregiving policy? First, there is clear evidence that the needs of homosexual families are discriminated against or ignored at all stages of the life course (Allen and Demo, 1995). Second, the current mood in politics, personified by the more conservative wing of the Republican party and the "Colorado for Family Values" campaign, denies the legitimacy of homosexual relationships and would not grant any public benefits to such arrangements on the grounds of the immorality of nonheterosexual liaisons. These two factors combine to suggest that it is unlikely that these relationships will be granted caregiving consideration and policy options in the near future.

When current Baby Boomers in such relationships begin to need care and public policy assistance, it is unclear what the state of public sentiment will then be. Currently, however, alternative caring arrangements have developed to deal with the special needs of homosexual elders and their families (Smith et al., 1995). For example, Slusher, Mayer, and Dunkle (1996), Kimmel (1992), and others show that older homosexuals have developed networks of caregiving among their homosexual friends in much the same way that childless elders rely more on friends. This scant research suggests that for those homosexuals who have maintained good relations with their families of procreation, these adult children provide care for their elderly parents just as heterosexual children do, and they can count on their parents in times of need as well. There is still not enough data on homosexual family life to generalize these findings, to give statistics on the size of the population for whom strong intergenerational ties are maintained, or to tell if children of homosexuals will come to the aid of their homosexual parents when they age. In absolute numbers, the size of the homosexual community engaged in parent-adult child caregiving may be relatively small when compared to other diverse caregiving situations.

A fifth variation in supportive arrangements that needs to be addressed is minority families. There are racial and ethnic variations in who composes the informal support system (Miller et al., 1996), as well as the household composition of the elderly in later life when care needs arise (De Vita, 1996). For example, two-parent households are more likely among Asians and Hispanics, births outside of marriage are highest among African-Americans (ibid.), and people of color are more likely than whites to live in extended, nontraditional family households (Chalfie, 1995). Each of these variations impact the likelihood of adult children turning to parents for assistance and the availability of adult children as caregivers in later life.

There is convincing evidence that minority families have different preferences and utilization patterns for informal and formal social support (Silverstein and Waite, 1993; Johnson, 1995). While the provision of informal support is related to less use of formal support among white, non-Hispanic families, among older African-Americans the availability of kin to help with informal support does not reduce the use of formal supports (Burton et al., 1995; Miner, 1995). Some of the early assumptions made by policymakers and service providers about minority culture and norms of family obligation and filial piety are not necessarily born out when formal service utilization patterns are considered in conjunction with the availability and use of informal family support (see the chapter by Villa in this volume). Moreover, program designs that are based on a white, middle-class family model will underserve minority populations or ignore them all together (Stoller and Gibson, 1994).

Last, family economic status impacts the ability of an aging family to deal with caregiving arrangements. The resources that high-income families will have to cope within caregiving situations will greatly overshadow the resources low-income families will have to call upon when caregiving needs arise. Issues of fairness surface when considering the diversity of family income, caregiving arrangements, and decisions about allocating public funds to help aging families. Many scholars and policymakers have pointed out that high-income families do not have the same level of need for public policy assistance as middle- or low-income families. For example, while a high-income family may need formal supportive services to be available in their communities, they may not need assistance in paying for such services. In contrast, middle- and low-income families may have such services available in their communities but may be unable to afford them or may not be poor enough to qualify for public assistance, such as Medicaid, to pay for them. Thus middle- and low-income families may rely on informal family care to a greater extent than high-income families because of the barrier that income places on their ability to purchase formal care. Ironically, these are the same families who may have the greatest need for formal community-based services so that they can juggle family and work obligations in order to stay "afloat."

Crucial for caregiving policy is the fact that older women living alone are at great risk for falling into poverty, especially if they have recently lost a spouse, gone through a divorce, never worked for pay, or are members of a minority group (see chapter by Steckenrider in this volume). These poor, older women are more likely than married women to need informal assistance from their families. Thus, income, marital status, and gender of an older individual have implications for the nuclear and extended family and the likelihood that they will be called upon for assistance.

Family Policies, Caregiving, and the Current Policy Environment

Decisions about who is "family" and who is responsible for the care of aging family members are made within the larger social and political context. The current trend (not unlike earlier times in America) is to hold families responsible for the primary care of their aging individual family members. While there is a high expectation of normative obligation to help older family members, evidence presented here suggests that there may be changes in the ability of adult children and family members to carry out this expectation because of changes within the actual structure of families, as well as changes in the labor force, the job market, and the diversity of care needs brought about by AIDS, drug dependency, and the aging of adult children with developmental disabilities and parents with Alzheimer's Disease. Future family caregiving behavior may not match policymakers' expectations of family responsibility.

These normative expectations of families exist in a policy environment in which government deficit reduction is a primary goal. Policymakers are focused on ways to cut spending and programs are viewed in terms of their expense (e.g., the Concord Coalition, 1993 and the Bipartisan Commission on Entitlement and Tax Reform, 1995). If a program to help caregivers assist their elders in the community was shown to cut expenses by delaying entry into a costly nursing home or reducing use of other formal services, then it might be expected to gain policy attention (for a recent cost estimate see Harrow, Tennstedt, and McKinlay, 1995). Moreover, as states are handed more power in the form of Medicaid waivers to find new alternatives to nursing home care, it also seems likely that states will look for less costly community-based services for the elderly. However, current proposals that either expect more of families or put more responsibility on families in the face of cuts in major federal programs for the elderly, are often made without establishing or funding the necessary community-based programs that need to be in place if they are to substitute for nursing home care (Estes and Swan, 1993).

Notably, some program spending increases have merely been slowed and these are technically not "cuts" to the programs. Slowing increases in spending on family programs may be viewed as ongoing support for such programs by some politicians, but the net result is that there is less money for the programs in the long run.

Some private companies have stepped in to aid families in the face of a changing balance between government and family responsibility for the elderly (Scharlach and Boyd, 1989; Seccombe, 1992). AT&T, Johnson & Johnson, Citicorp, and Exxon, for example, are part of the American Business Collaboration for Quality Dependent Care, a business consortium whose goal is to establish eldercare programs for employees in caregiving situations (Gilpin, 1995).

However, while these programs offer alternatives to government-sponsored solutions, many have not been highly utilized and do not offer the types of services that families often need. Their success in the future remains to be seen.

While many alternative family forms exist, few alternatives to the traditional family model are recognized or legitimated by policy (Chalfie, 1995). This means that not all families are helped equally by policy efforts and thus must seek out alternatives to public assistance with caregiving. The current political environment does not suggest much tolerance for recognizing alternative supportive arrangements other than the nuclear, heterosexual family model. Indeed, some would argue that homosexual families and cohabitating families are not "families" at all, instead they are living arrangements that cannot perform the same functions as a stable family unit (e.g., Popenoe, 1994).

Three things are true for the future: (1) more aging families will be facing the dilemmas raised by caregiving situations; (2) the needs of an aging population will continue to rise at a time when many Baby Boomer adult children are faced with their own aging, instability in employment situations, and low savings; and (3) the complexity of family care arrangements and caregiving needs will increase rather than become more simplified as family demographics change.

Proposals

Given the current policy environment, several policy solutions for aging families and their caregiving needs seem possible. First, it is reasonable to expect that there will be more need for community-based services if there is more responsibility being placed on families for care arrangements. Thus, more accessible community-based care options are needed. In particular, health care, personal care, and household services have been found to be the most beneficial for lessening the negative consequences of caregiving, such as stress, depression, and isolation experienced by family caregivers (Bass, Noelker, and Rechlin, 1996). But making such services widely available will not be enough. The services must be made affordable for low- and moderate-income families either through a sliding-scale fee or through targeting of public assistance resources.

Second, more options for job flexibility are needed and private employer assistance with and support of eldercare should be encouraged. The greater the support of employers for caregiving employees, the greater the likelihood that families will have resources to pay for services on their own rather than relying on government assistance. Moreover, there is evidence accumulating that suggests that eldercare programs are less costly to employers than is employee turnover due to caregiving responsibilities, and that such programs reduce work-family conflicts and stress among caregivers and improve their performance on the job (Barr, Johnson, and Warshaw, 1992).

Third, more policy attention needs to be directed toward the needs of families facing unusual caregiving dilemmas such as families where grandparents have become caregivers for grandchildren or for their sick or disabled adult children. In these situations, aging family members are much more vulnerable to a variety of social and economic problems that exceed the current range of caregiving support options. Pillemer (1996), in a review of recent works on caregiving, persuasively argued that not all caregivers may need assistance by means of a caregiving policy, and he pointed out that caregiving researchers have shown that about two-thirds of family caregivers do not experience any burden, burnout, or stress. Pillemer provocatively raises the issue of why researchers and policymakers are trying to help these family members who are managing on their own. Perhaps the best targets for caregiving and eldercare programs are those families with special considerations, such as the diversity of care arrangements identified in this chapter.

Fourth, nontraditional family forms exist, whether their needs and their status as a "family" are recognized through public policy or not. If the current trend in government is not to extend policy support to these family forms directly, it is necessary to sensitize service providers and formal caregivers so that they recognize these hidden care arrangements and begin to develop their own principles and policies for nonkin supportive situations. Moreover, equity concerns would warrant a reconsideration of public benefit eligibility rules so that, in efforts to deny benefits to nontraditional family forms, policymakers do not end up actually giving an advantage to nonrelated individuals providing care at the expense of related but nontraditional caregivers (see Chalfie, 1995).

Fifth, and last, families change over time and their needs change as well. A constant evaluation of policies and needs should occur, especially in light of the changes in family demographics and in the diversity of care arrangements. Old models of care and assumptions about family life may be incorrect and should be tested as the Baby Boomers age and bring with them a whole range of diverse family forms and caregiving needs. Research should clarify which family caregiver assistance programs are most beneficial to which caregivers and why (Pillemer, 1996), and there needs to be more evaluation of family care in terms of its quality (Kane and Penrod, 1995) as well as the reasons why it does not become a stressor or negative experience for all family caregivers.

There is room for innovation in policy options as well as opportunities for creative private solutions during this particular period of government retrenchment and devolution. Rather than taking a doom-and-gloom approach to the current political circumstances, it would seem wise for those concerned about family caregiving to use this as a period of reevaluation and redirection of resources to address the current and future needs of our aging families.

References

Ahlburg, D. A., and De Vita, C. J. (1992). New realities of the American family. *Population Bulletin*, 47(2). Washington, DC: Population Reference Bureau.

Allen, K. R., and Demo, D. H. (1995). The families of lesbians and gay men: A new frontier in family research. *Journal of Marriage and the Family*, 57, 111–27.

Allen, S. M. (1994). Gender differences in spousal caregiving and unmet need for care. *Journal of Gerontology: Social Sciences*, 49, S187–S195.

Barr, J. K., Johnson, K. W., and Warshaw, L. J. (1992). Supporting the elderly: Workplace programs for employed caregivers. *Milbank Quarterly*, 70, 509–33.

Bass, D. M., Noelker, L. S., and Rechlin, L. R. (1996). The moderating influence of service use on negative caregiving consequences. *Journal of Gerontology: Social Sciences*, 51B, S121–S131.

Bedford, V. H. (1995). Sibling relationships in middle and old age. In R. Blieszner and V. H. Bedford (Eds.), *Handbook of Aging and the Family*, pp. 201–22. Westport, CT: Greenwood Press.

Bengtson, V. L., Rosenthal, C., and Burton, L. (1990). Families and aging: Diversity and heterogeneity. In R. Binstock and L. George (Eds.), *Handbook of Aging and the Social Sciences, Third Edition*, pp. 263–87. New York: Academic.

———. (1996). Paradoxes of families and aging. In R. Binstock and L. George (Eds.), *Handbook of Aging and the Social Sciences, 4th ed.*, pp. 254–82. New York: Academic.

Bipartisan Commission on Entitlement and Tax Reform. (1995). *Final Report to the President.* Washington, DC: Government Printing Office.

Bouvier, L. F., and De Vita, C.J. (1991). The Baby Boom—Entering Midlife. *Population Bulletin*, 46(3). Washington, DC: Population Reference Bureau.

Bradsher, J. E., Estes, C. L., and Stuart, M. H. (1995). Adult day care: A fragmented system of policy and funding streams. *Journal of Aging and Social Policy*, 7, 17–38.

Brody, E. M. (1990). *Women in the Middle: Their Parent-Care Years.* New York: Springer.

———; Litvin, S. J., Albert, S. M., and Hoffman, C. J. (1994). Marital status of daughters and patterns of parent care. *Journal of Gerontology: Social Sciences*, 49, S95–S103.

Bulcroft, K. A., and Bulcroft, R.A. (1991). The timing of divorce: Effects on parent-child relationships in later life. *Research on Aging*, 13, 226–43.

Bulcroft, K. A., Van Leynseele, J., and Borgatta, E. F. (1989). Filial responsibility laws: Issues and state statutes. *Research on Aging*, 11, 374–93.

Burton, L., Kasper, J., Shore, A., Cagney, K., La Veist, T., Cubbin, C., and German, P. (1995). The structure of informal care: Are there differences by race? *Gerontologist*, 35, 744–52.

Cantor, M. H. (1983). Strain among caregivers: A study of experience in the United States. *Gerontologist*, 26, 597–604.

Chalfie, D. (1994). *Going It Alone: A Closer Look at Grandparents Parenting Grandchildren.* Washington, DC: American Association of Retired Persons Women's Initiative.

———. (1995). *The Real Golden Girls: The Prevalence and Policy Treatment of Midlife and Older People Living in Nontraditional Households.* Washington, DC: American Association of Retired Persons Women's Initiative.

Cicirelli, V. G. (1983). A comparison of helping behavior to elderly parents of adult children with intact and disrupted marriages. *Gerontologist*, 23, 619–25.

Concord Coalition. (1993). *The Zero Deficit Plan.* Washington, DC: Concord Coalition.

Connidis, I. A. (1994). Sibling support in older age. *Journal of Gerontology: Social Sciences*, 9, S309–S317.

Cooney, T. M., and Uhlenberg, P. (1990). The role of divorce in men's relations with their adult children after mid-life. *Journal of Marriage and the Family*, 52, 677–88.

De Vita, D. J. (1996). The United States at mid-decade. *Population Bulletin*, 50(4). Washington, DC: Population Reference Bureau.

Doty, P. (1986). Family care: The role of public policy. *Milbank Quarterly*, 64, 34–75.

Ernst, R. L., and Hay, J. W. (1994). The U.S. economic and social costs of Alzheimer's Disease revisited. *American Journal of Public Health*, 84, 1261–64.

Estes, C. L., and Swan, J. H. (1993). *The Long Term Care Crisis: Elders Trapped in the No-Care Zone*. Newbury Park, CA: Sage.

Finley, N. J., Roberts, M. D., and Banahan, B. F. (1988). Motivations and inhibitors of attitudes of filial obligation toward aging parents. *Gerontologist*, 28, 73–78.

Genevay, B. (1993). "Creating" families: Older people alone. In Linda Burton (Ed.), *Families and Aging*, pp. 121–27. Amityville, NY: Baywood Publishing.

George, L. K., and Gwyther, L. P. (1986). Caregiver well-being: A multidimensional examination of the family caregivers of demented adults. *Gerontologist*, 26, 253–59.

Gerald, L. B. (1993). Paid family caregiving: A review of progress and policies. In S. A. Bass and R. Morris (Eds.), *International Perspectives on State and Family Support for the Elderly*, pp. 73–89. New York: Haworth Press.

Gilpin, K. N. (1995). Dependent-care aid for employees at 21 companies. *New York Times*, 14 September, p. D4.

Gottlieb, B. H., Kelloway, E. K., and Fraboni, M. (1994). Aspects of eldercare that place employees at risk. *Gerontologist*, 34, 815–21.

Harrow, B. S., Tennstedt, S. L., and McKinlay, J. B. (1995). How costly is it to care for disabled elders in a community setting? *Gerontologist*, 35, 803–13.

Hodgson, L. G. (1992). Adult grandchildren and their grandparents: The enduring bond. *International Journal of Aging and Human Development*, 34, 209–25.

———. and Cutler, S. J. (1994). Caregiving and Alzheimer's Disease. *Educational Gerontology*, 20, 665–78.

Hooyman, N. R. (1992). Social policies and gender inequities in caregiving. In J. W. Dwyer and R. T. Coward (Eds.), *Gender, Families, and Elder Care*, pp. 181–201. Newbury Park, CA: Sage.

Hu, T., Huang, L., and Cartwright, W. (1986). Evaluation of the costs of caring for the senile demented elderly: A pilot study. *Gerontologist*, 26, 158–63.

Jendrek, M. P. (1993). Grandparents who parent their grandchildren: Effects on lifestyle. *Journal of Marriage and the Family*, 55, 609–21.

Johnson, C. L. (1993). Divorced and reconstituted families: Effects on the older generation. In Linda Burton (Ed.), *Families and Aging*, pp. 33–41. Amityville, NY: Baywood Publishing.

———. (1995). Cultural diversity in the late-life family. In R. Blieszner and V. H. Bedford (Eds.), *Handbook of Aging and the Family*, pp. 307–31. Westport, CT: Greenwood Press.

Kane, R. A., and Penrod, J. D. (Eds.) (1995). *Family Caregiving in an Aging Society: Policy Perspectives*. Newbury Park, CA: Sage.

Kimmel, D. C. (1992). The families of older gay men and lesbians. *Generations*, 16, 37–38.

Kingson, E., and O'Grady-LeShane, R. (1993). The effects of caregiving on women's Social Security benefits. *Gerontologist*, 33, 230–39.

Lawton, L., Silverstein, M., and Bengtson, V. L. (1994a). Closeness, contact and commitment between generations. In V. L. Bengtson and R. A. Harootyan (Eds.), *Intergenerational Linkages: Hidden Connections in American Society*, pp. 19–42. New York: Springer.

———. (1994b). Affection, social contact, and geographic distance between adult children and their parents. *Journal of Marriage and the Family*, 56, 57–68.

Lee, G. R., Dwyer, J. W., and Coward, R. T. (1993). Gender differences in parent care: Demographic factors and same-gender preferences. *Journals of Gerontology: Social Sciences*, 48, S9–S16.

Liebig, P. S. (1993). The effects of federalism on policies for care of the aged in Canada and the United States. In S. A. Bass and R. Morris (Eds.), *International Perspectives on State and Family Support for the Elderly*, pp. 13–37. New York: Haworth Press.

Linsk, N. L., Keigher, S. M., Simon-Rusinowitz, L., and England, S. E. (1992). *Wages for Caring: Compensating Family Care of the Elderly*. New York: Praeger Publishing.

Matthews, S. H. (1992). Gender and the division of filial responsibility between lone sisters and their brothers. *Journal of Gerontology: Social Sciences,* 50B, S312–S320.

Miller, B., Campbell, R. T., Davis, L., Furner, S., Giachello, A., Prohaska, T., Kaufman, J. E., Li, M., and Perez, C. (1996). Minority use of community long-term care services: A comparative analysis. *Journal of Gerontology: Social Sciences,* 51B, S70–S81.

Miner, S. (1995). Racial differences in family support and formal service utilization among older persons: A nonrecursive model. *Journal of Gerontology: Social Sciences,* 50B, S143–S153.

Minkler, M., Roe, K. M., and Price, M. (1992). The physical and emotional health of grandmothers raising grandchildren in the crack cocaine epidemic. *Gerontologist,* 32, 752–61.

Moen, P., and Forest, K.B. (1995). Family policies for an aging society: Moving to the Twenty-First Century. *Gerontologist,* 35, 825–30.

Moen, P., Robison, J., and Fields, V. (1994). Women's work and caregiving roles: A life course approach. *Journal of Gerontology: Social Sciences,* 49, S176–S186.

Moen, P., and Schorr, A. L. (1988). Families and social policy. In M. B. Sussman and S. K. Steinmetz (Eds.), *Handbook of Marriage and the Family,* pp. 795–813. New York: Plenum Press.

Mullen, F. (1995). *A Tangled Web: Public Benefits, Grandparents, and Grandchildren.* Public Policy Institute Report no. 9502. Washington, DC: American Association of Retired Persons.

Myers, G. C. (1992). Demographic aging and family support for older persons. In H. L. Kendig, A. Hashimoto, and L. C. Coppard (Eds.), *Family Support for the Elderly: The International Experience,* pp. 31–68. New York: Oxford University Press.

Pillemer, K. (1996). Family caregiving: What would a martian say? Book review. *Gerontologist,* 36, 269–71.

Popenoe, D. (1994). The family condition: Cultural change and public policy. In H. J. Aaron, T. E. Mann, and T. Taylor (Eds.), *Values and Public Policy,* pp. 81–112. Washington, DC: Brookings Institution.

Presser, H. B. (1989). Some economic complexities of child care provided by grandmothers. *Journal of Marriage and the Family,* 51, 581–91.

Robertson, J. F. (1995). Grandparenting in an era of rapid change. In R. Blieszner and V. H. Bedford (Eds.), *Handbook of Aging and the Family,* pp. 243–60. Westport, CT: Greenwood Press.

Robison, J., Moen, P., and Dempster-McClain, D. (1995). Women's caregiving: Changing profiles and pathways. *Journal of Gerontology: Social Sciences*, 50B, S362–S373.

Scharlach, A. E., and Boyd, S. L. (1989). Caregiving and employment: Results of an employee survey. *Gerontologist*, 29, 382–387.

Scharlach, A. E., Lowe, B. F., and Schneider, E. L. (1991). *Eldercare and the Workforce: Blueprint for Action.* Toronto, Canada: Lexington Books.

Seccombe, K. (1992). Employment, the family, and employer-based policies. In J. W. Dwyer and R. T. Coward (Eds.), *Gender, Families, and Elder Care*, pp. 165–80. Newbury Park, CA: Sage.

Shanas, E. (1979). The family as a social support system in old age. *Gerontologist*, 19, 169–74.

Shank, S. E. (1988). Women and the labor market: The link grows stronger. *Monthly Labor Review*, 3, 3–8.

Silverstein, M., and Waite, L. J. (1993). Are Blacks more likely than whites to receive and provide social support in middle and old age? Yes, no, and maybe so. *Journal of Gerontology: Social Sciences*, 48, S212–S222.

Slusher, M. P., Mayer, C. J., and Dunkle, R.E. (1996). Gays and Lesbians Older and Wiser (GLOW): A support group for older gay people. *Gerontologist*, 36, 118–23.

Smith, G. C., Tobin, S. S., Robertson-Tchabo, E. A., and Power, P. W. (Eds.) (1995). *Strengthening Aging Families: Diversity in Practice and Policy.* Newbury Park, CA: Sage.

Spitze, G., Logan, J. R., Deane, G., and Zerger, S. (1994). Adult children's divorce and intergenerational relationships. *Journal of Marriage and the Family*, 56, 279–93.

Starrels, M. E., Ingersoll-Dayton, B., Neal, M. B., and Yamada, H. (1995). Intergenerational solidarity and the workplace: Employees' caregiving for their parents. *Journal of Marriage and the Family*, 57, 751–62.

Stephens, A. P., and Franks, M. M. (1995). Spillover between daughters' roles as caregiver and wife: Interference or enhancement? *Journal of Gerontology: Psychological Sciences*, 50B, P9–P17.

Stoller, E. P., and Gibson, R. C. (1994). *Worlds of Difference: Inequality in the Aging Experience.* Thousand Oaks, CA: Pine Forge Press.

Stone, R., Cafferata, G. L., and Sangl, J. (1987). Caregivers of the frail elderly: A national profile. *Gerontologist*, 26, 616–26.

Stone, R., and Kemper, P. (1989). Spouses and children of disabled elders: How large a constituency for long-term care reform? *Milbank Quarterly*, 67, 485–505.

Sutton, E. (Ed.) (1993). *Older Adults with Developmental Disabilities: Optimizing Choice and Change*. Baltimore, MD: Paul H. Brookes Publishing.

Thomas, J. L. (1993). Concerns regarding adult children's assistance: A comparison of young-old and old-old parents. *Journal of Gerontology: Social Sciences*, 48, S315–S322.

Treas, J. (1995). Older Americans in the 1990s and beyond. *Population Bulletin*, 50 (2). Washington, DC: Population Reference Bureau.

Uhlenberg, P. (1980). Death and the family. *Journal of Family History*, fall, 313–20.

———. (1993). Demographic change and kin relationships in later life. In G. L. Maddox and M. P. Lawton (Eds.), *Annual Review of Gerontology and Geriatrics, Vol. 13, Focus on Kinship, Aging, and Social Change*, pp. 219–38. New York: Springer.

———, Cooney, T. M., and Boyd, R. (1990). Divorce for women after midlife. *Journal of Gerontology: Social Sciences*, 45, S3–S11.

U.S. Department of Labor. (1993). *Compliance Guide to the Family Medical and Leave Act*. Washington, DC: White House Publication 1421.

White-Means, S., and Chollet, D. (1996). Opportunity wages and workforce adjustments: Understanding the cost of in-home elder care. *Journal of Gerontology: Social Sciences*, 51B, S82–S90.

Wolfson, S. L., Handfield-Jones, Glass, K. C., McClaran, J., and Keyserlingk, E. (1993). Adult children's perceptions of their responsibility to provide care for dependent elderly parents. *Gerontologist*, 33, 315–23.

Wright, L. K., Clipp, E. C., and George, L. K. (1993). Health consequences of caregiver stress. *Medicine, Exercise, Nutrition, and Health*, 2, 181–95.

Zimmerman, S. L. (1988). *Understanding Family Policy: Theoretical Approaches*. Newbury Park, CA: Sage.

Chapter 11   *Re-read if time Permits* (handwritten)

Aging Policy and the Experience of Older Minorities

VALENTINE M. VILLA

Diversity and the Elderly Population

As we enter the twenty-first Century and witness an unprecedented growth in the elderly population, we will also witness an increase in their diversity. In 1990, 13% of the 32 million Americans aged 65 and over were members of a minority group, by the year 2030 Census Bureau projections indicate that 25% of the elderly population will be minorities (American Association of Retired Persons, 1994). Between 1990 and 2030, the white non-Hispanic population aged 65 and over is expected to increase 93%, whereas the older minority population is expected to increase by 328%, with the number of African-American elders tripling, and Asian, Hispanic, and Native American elders increasing by 693%, 555%, and 231% respectively (ibid., 1994).

The growth in the minority elderly population and the increasing diversity among those over age 65 challenges us to investigate the applicability of existing and proposed programs and policies for the elderly (Markides and Mindel, 1987; Burton, Dilworth-Anderson, and Bengston, 1991). Designing policies that are more responsive to the needs of a growing diverse older adult population, increasingly composed of members of minorities, will require that we consider how race, immigration, language, economic status, gender, and historical experiences influence the aging process (Stanford and Torres-Gil, 1991). In addition, the fiscal constraints faced by many aging programs will continue to underscore the importance of incorporating diversity in program

planning and development in order to target needs among the elderly population more appropriately and efficiently (Mui and
Burnette, 1994). To achieve more efficient and effective policies and
programs, those that better dovetail with the needs of the older
adult population, we must broaden our knowledge of the aging
process of all groups in society (Andersen, 1993). To this end, after
a review of the relevance of race, ethnicity, and minority group
membership for the study of aging and aging policy, this chapter
addresses the potential effect of three policy issues on minority
elders and provides recommendations for the design of aging policies and programs that better fit the aging experiences of current
and future older minorities.

The Relevance of Race and Ethnicity for the Study of Aging and Aging Policy

The relevance of race and ethnicity for the study of aging and
aging policy is more than a matter of demographics. Investigation
of the minority aging experience is pertinent for the following reasons: (1) the differential impact that aging policy has on minority
group members (Calasanti, 1996); (2) empirical evidence that indicates that older minority populations have higher rates of poverty
and experience poorer health relative to non-Hispanic whites
(Gerontological Society of America, 1994); and (3) the impact that
racism, segregation, and oppression, often experienced by minority
group members, have on their life choices and opportunities, mental and physical health, and, life course trajectory (Bayne-Smith,
1996; Applewhite and Daley, 1988; Stoller and Gibson, 1994).

To suggest that the minority elderly population is a homog-
enous group would be erroneous. Older minorities constitute a
number of different racial and ethnic groups with distinct cultures,
languages, and migration histories (Sotomayor, 1993). However,
there are certain issues that disproportionately affect minority elderly populations, including poverty and poor health (Chen, 1994;
Markides and Black, 1996; Mutchler and Burr, 1991; Sotomayor,
1993). According to Krause and Wray (1991: 25), "a look beyond the
mean illustrates that minority elderly remain among the most
economically disadvantaged and chronically ill in society, and most
in need of social support and health services."

Differential Impact of Aging Policy

While policies regarding services, benefits, and eligibility for
aging programs affect all older adults, the impact of these policies

differs by race and ethnicity. For example, Calasanti (1996) argues that while retirement and income policies and programs such as Social Security create barriers and opportunities for all older workers, both the form and extent of their impact varies across groups. Social Security legislation assumes stable work histories and the availability of other sources of retirement income such as private pensions, savings, and investments. These patterns are most characteristic of the experience of white males (ibid.; see chapter by Steckenrider in this volume). In contrast, the work histories of many minorities are characterized by sporadic employment and concentration in "junk jobs" (Esping-Andersen, 1990). Junk jobs refers to low-paying jobs that are primarily in the service industry that offer no benefits or pensions.

Indeed, there is recent evidence that pension levels have dropped among African-Americans and Hispanics over the past 15 years. According to Chen (1994), the percentage of African Americans covered by private pensions dropped from 45.1% in 1979 to 33.8% in 1993, and coverage among Hispanics dropped from 37.7% to 24.6%. Instead, minority elderly populations are more reliant on Social Security for income in old age (Garcia, 1993; Stanford, Torres-Gil, and Schoenrock, 1990; John, 1990) because they are more likely to be poor or have low incomes in retirement compared to nonminority populations (Chen, 1994). According to Garcia (1990), Social Security accounts for 56% of income for African-Americans, 51% for Hispanic elderly, and 39% for white elderly. Data for Native Americans reveal that over 50% rely on Social Security as their sole source of income and 15% rely on Supplemental Security Income (SSI) as their sole source of income (John, 1994).

Proposed options for reforming the Social Security system, such as those that call for changing the fundamental structure of the program, will heavily impact minority populations who are more reliant on Social Security and less likely to have savings and/ or other pensions. One proposal recently put forth by the Advisory Council on Social Security (1997) aims to privatize the program by creating Personal Security Accounts (PSA). Under PSAs, workers would invest 5% of their income under the Social Security wage base in a personal security account that they would individually own and privately manage by picking stocks and bonds for investment. The remaining 7.4% in income paid to Social Security in taxes would be allocated to the Social Security trust fund. Upon retirement each retiree would receive $410 a month, plus whatever money they earned in their individual investment account.

Critics of privatization argue that economic security will depend on an individual's prowess in selecting the "right" investment, and, while perhaps some retirees would do better, others may lose all of their money through poor investments. This would mean a decline in retirement savings (Kingson and Quadagno, 1995), and an increase in economic vulnerability. Kingson and Quadagno argue that proposals for reforming Social Security, such as privatization, ignore the human consequences that these changes will have particularly for low-income populations, women, and minorities who are more heavily dependent on the program for security in old age. It is estimated that Social Security provides 75% of the aggregate income of older households with annual income less than $10,000, compared to 31% for households with average incomes above $30,000. In addition, among the population over age 65, 62% receive at least half of their income from Social Security (Aleska, 1994)—many of these individuals are members of minority populations. Garcia (1993) estimates that while 23% of older Hispanics are in poverty, an additional 37% would fall below the poverty level if it were not for Social Security. Thus, given the extent to which minority elders rely on Social Security, it is clearly an important floor of protection against poverty for minority populations; changes in its basic structure should be carefully considered.

Health and Economic Status of Minority Elders

Investigations of the health status of the elderly population reveal that while there has been a general improvement in their health as a whole, the situation for minority elders has not kept pace (Gerontological Society of America, 1994). In spite of general improvement in mortality and morbidity among the older adult population, minority elders still display disadvantages in certain diseases and in physical functioning (Johnson and Wolinsky, 1994; Markides and Black, 1996; Mutchler and Burr, 1991; Jackson, 1988; Villa, Lubben, and Moon, 1995). There also is evidence that these disadvantages persist even when socioeconomic status is held constant (Mutchler and Burr, 1991; Ferraro, 1987; Krause, 1987).

Specifically, older Hispanics are disadvantaged relative to non-Hispanic whites for certain chronic diseases, most notably diabetes. Mexican-Americans have a prevalence rate for noninsulin dependent diabetes two to five times greater than among the general U.S. population in both sexes and at every age (Perez-Stable, McMillan, and Harris, 1989; Hanis et al., 1983; Stern et al., 1983) and there is much higher mortality from diabetes among Hispanics compared to

African-Americans and whites at every age and for both sexes (Stern and Gaskill, 1978; Bradshaw and Foner, 1978). In addition, older Hispanics experience more bed disability days, restricted activity days, and difficulty with activities of daily living (Markides, Coreil, and Rogers, 1989; Markides and Mindel, 1987; Markides and Martin, 1983; Markides and Lee, 1990; O'Donnel, 1989; Commonwealth Fund Commission Report, 1989; National Center for Health Statistics, 1984; Cantor and Mayer, 1976; Newquist, 1976).

Like Hispanics, African-American elders are disadvantaged relative to whites for a number of disease conditions and are more likely to be "less healthy" and experience limitations in activity due to poor health (Markides and Black, 1996). Data for older African-Americans indicate that the prevalence for chronic disease is twice as high as among whites (Waller, 1989) and the impact of certain diseases such as hypertension on disability is greater for African-American males than for white males (Johnson and Wolinsky, 1994).

Explanations for disadvantages in health experienced by minority elders have primarily focused on the role of socioeconomic status. The link between poor health and low socioeconomic status has been well documented (Kaplan et al., 1987; Williams, 1990) and it has been suggested that the disproportionate poor health among older minorities is related to their higher levels of poverty and low income (Kiyak and Hooyman,1994). Despite the dramatic improvement in the economic well-being of the population aged 65 and over since the 1960s, pockets of poverty persist primarily among ethnic minority men and women (Garcia, 1990; Kiyak and Hooyman, 1994). In 1990, the poverty rate for elderly whites was 10.1%, 12.2% for Asians, 22.5% for Hispanics, and 33.8% for African-Americans (U.S. Bureau of the Census, 1990). Data on Native Americans reveal that 72% of elderly women and 50% of elderly men are in poverty (John, 1990). In addition, low-income minority elderly populations have low education levels that are related to economic disadvantage and poor health. In examining education differentials, Taeuber (1992) found that 57% of older African-Americans and 64% of older Hispanics have less than eight years of schooling compared to 30% of white elders. Furthering our knowledge of the link between socioeconomic status and poor health across the life course is "badly needed," and is essential in advancing our understanding of health differentials between minority and non-Hispanic white populations (Markides and Black, 1996).

Evidence to date suggests that policy proposals such as the changes occurring in welfare and Medicaid programs have not taken into consideration the impact these changes will have on the health and well-being of minorities. For example, the Personal Responsibility and Work Opportunity Reconciliation Act signed into law by President Clinton in August 1996, limits eligibility and reduces payment levels under SSI, thereby not only removing and/or reducing a floor of income for elderly poor, many of whom are minorities, but also limiting their access to Medicaid that is affected by eligibility for SSI. Furthermore, changes under Medicaid proposed by Clinton and Congress that call for capping spending and block granting Medicaid to the states have the potential to limit access to health and long-term care for low-income minority populations. To reduce the rate of growth in expenditures under Medicaid, states will probably rely on traditional methods of cost control. Strategies for controlling spending include restricting eligibility, reimbursement, covered services, and quality standards (Wiener, 1996). The problem with these strategies is that they limit access to services and have the potential to seriously reduce quality of care (ibid.). If states are no longer held accountable for mandatory services, a wide array of service reductions and elimination of services can be expected (Riley, 1995). At risk will be low income and minority populations that are disproportionately reliant on Medicaid for basic health care and as a supplement to out- of-pocket costs under Medicare.

The Impact of Racism, Segregation, and Oppression

Understanding the minority aging experience also requires acknowledging the social-structural barriers such as racism, oppression, and segregation experienced by minority group members. These constraints are associated with economic disadvantage and they limit opportunities and choice across the life course and negatively impact physical and mental health status (Stoller and Gibson, 1994). According to Kiyak and Hooyman (1994), structural factors underlying high poverty rates among older minorities include life-long discrimination in employment and education resulting in low levels of education and high levels of unemployment and underemployment across the life course. Moreover, there are multiple ways in which discrimination encountered throughout life translates into an accumulation of disadvantage in old age. Stoller and Gibson (1994) maintain that there is little doubt that legally segregated school systems and legally sanctioned discriminatory hiring practices limited the opportunity of today's elderly African-Americans in accumulating wealth and financial assets over their life course.

Indeed, Bayne-Smith (1996) argues that American society is essentially stratified by race and that the resulting deprivation limits the capacity of nonwhites to function not only within the economic system, but also within the remaining structures and institutions of society.

Furthermore, it has been argued that observed health differences between minority populations and non-Hispanic whites are not only the result of socioeconomic status and poverty, but are also the result of race, or, more aptly, the American response to race and people of color. In short, race in the United States accounts for health differences because race is a pervasive issue that affects every area of life. The effects of racism on the health of minority populations is perhaps most clearly manifested in limited access to health and social services. The segregation associated with race and minority group membership contributes to the lack of health care services in minority communities, even when they are middle class (Bayne-Smith, 1996). The indirect effects of racism on health are also apparent when one considers the impact of racism on mental health and well-being. The lack of group respect accorded to minority populations can impact mental health and negatively affect feelings of self-worth and self-esteem (Applewhite and Daley, 1988; Bayne-Smith, 1996), and can lead to the proliferation of "unhealthy" behaviors among minority group members as a means of coping. According to Bayne-Smith (1996:14), health-related nihilistic behavior among minority group members is "in many respects, a response to recalcitrant racism in the United States that often subjects members of racial minorities to a lived experience of coping with horrifying meaninglessness and hopelessness." Clearly, if we are to design and develop policies that better the lives of the older population we must be aware of the impact these issues have on the lives of minorities over the life course.

What is disheartening, however, is that much of the knowledge about the effect of racism, segregation, and oppression is not new. From a national perspective, these are issues that have been grappled with for decades. At points in history, there were moments of forward movement, such as the civil rights laws, but more recently the shift seems to be backward with state level attempts to do away with affirmative action, changes in federal law regarding the treatment of minorities in the awarding of federal contracts, and the anti-immigrant wave of the 1990s. This all suggests that many Americans perceive the negative effects of racism to be overcome.

Aging Policy Issues and the Minority Elderly

Improving the experience of minority populations and our knowledge of the aging experience of older minorities requires examination of the potential impact that policies, programs, and legislation have on their health, economic, and social well-being. Understanding the experience of oppressed groups shifts our focus to policies that we might otherwise ignore (Calasanti, 1996). The following section examines the effect of cost containment proposals, access and acceptability of aging services among minority populations, and the effect of anti-immigrant legislation.

here

Cost Containment and Minority Elders

One area of health policy recently receiving considerable attention is cost containment. Over the past few years numerous proposals have been generated for curtailing the costs of aging programs, especially the costs of Medicare and Medicaid (Villers Foundation, 1987; see chapter by Binstock in this volume). Cost containment in Medicare, Medicaid, and the Older Americans Act programs was perhaps most clearly articulated and popularized in the 1994 Republican congressional platform, "Contract with America." Under the contract, premiums, out-of-pocket costs, and deductibles under Medicare would have doubled, and Medicaid cost sharing would have increased with states having the option of limiting the amount and scope of assistance provided to Medicaid recipients (e.g., eliminate protection for spousal impoverishment, coverage for out-of-pocket costs under Medicare for the poor, and adoption of third-party liability) (Administration on Aging, 1995). Increased spending by the elderly for services and cost containment policy in general have the potential to increase economic vulnerability among minority elders and to decrease their access to health and long-term care services because of their inability to afford additional costs.

Cost containment policies that pose added costs to consumers are particularly troubling because of the lack of insurance coverage among minority populations. Health insurance coverage among older adults also reveals a disadvantage among minorities. While 75% of the total population aged 65 and over have private supplemental insurance and only 15% rely on Medicare as their sole source of insurance, 13% of non-Hispanic whites rely solely on Medicare, as compared to 36.2% of older African-Americans and 31.6% of Hispanic elders (National Center for Health Statistics, 1995). While 79% of older non-Hispanic whites have both Medicare and supplemental insurance, only 43.6% of African-American elders and 38.1% of Hispanic elders have both. Furthermore, 4.2% of non-Hispanic whites have Medicare and Medicaid, and 13.3% of older African-Americans and 23.6% of older Hispanics receive both Medicare and Medicaid. It is estimated that low-income Hispanics currently spend 29% of their annual income on out-of-pocket costs for health care compared to 21% for all older Americans (Sotomayor, 1993). Indeed, drastic cuts to Medicaid, lack of coverage for Medicare premiums, and increased cost sharing under Medicaid will leave many elderly minorities who cannot afford these out-of-pocket costs without coverage for health and long-term care services.

Other strategies aimed at cost containment include granting states waivers under Medicaid to shift Medicaid recipients into managed care systems. While proponents of managed care systems maintain that they have been effective at containing health care costs because of their emphasis on cost containment, it is not clear whether this is due to increased efficiency, or whether those initially in better health are more likely to join managed care systems. There has been a tendency for large capitated systems to "skim" the healthiest patients who will be lower service users, and to avoid the chronically ill and disabled who are more likely to be low income and members of minority populations. Therefore, the services offered under managed care arrangements typically do not mesh well with services needed by minority populations, for instance, ongoing diabetes management. Therefore, because managed care is structured as a medical gate-keeper rather than an advocate, traditionally underserved populations like the low-income and minority groups are at risk of continuing to be underserved even when covered (Wallace and Villa, forthcoming).

Limited access to health and long-term care services for older minorities means that greater responsibility for their well-being will be shifted to minority families who, like their elderly members, are economically and socially vulnerable. The median family income for Mexican- Americans in 1990 was $23,400 compared to $35,200 for the total population, and 28% of Hispanic families were living below the poverty line, more than double the total population rate of 12.8% (U.S. Bureau of the Census, 1992). According to the Center on Budget and Policy Priorities (1989), about one in four Hispanic workers paid by the hour does not earn enough to keep a family of three out of poverty. Morrison (1990) found that the median income for African-American families in 1987 was $18,100, which represents 56% of the median family income for white families ($32,270). This proportion has not changed since 1979 and the median income levels for both African-American and Hispanic families in 1987 was not significantly different (after adjusting for inflation) from what it was in 1979. In addition, among African-Americans and Hispanics there is a high ratio of female-headed households resulting in more reliance on single-parent income and an increase in the number of families living in poverty (National Research Council, 1989; Garcia, 1993).

Increases in teen pregnancy and in the prevalence of AIDS and HIV among younger members of minority populations have resulted in an increase in four-generation households where middle-aged women are caring for their parents, adult children, and grandchildren (National Council of La Raza, 1992; Antonnucci and Cantor, 1994; Sotomayor, 1993). Accordingly, there is an increasing number of minority women aged 55 and over who must quit their jobs to care for family members, while at the same time receive no income from Social Security or private pensions (Garcia, 1993). Clearly, minority families have accepted the "responsibility" of caring for family members and indeed express a preference for caring for relatives in the home (Kiyak and Hooyman, 1994; Antonucci and Cantor, 1994). But, given the above challenges, caring for family members without some public assistance is unrealistic (see chapter by Parrott in this volume).

Access and Acceptability of Community and In-home Services

For minority elders to benefit from in-home and community-based services, their access to these programs must be improved. Investigation of service use among minorities reveals that participation rates are lower than needs would indicate (Damron-Rodriquez, Wallace, and Kington, 1994; Hyde and Torres-Gil, 1991). Studies of utilization find that despite difficulties with activities of daily living and disabilities associated with chronic conditions, older minorities are more likely to use informal support than formal supportive services. An analysis of health and service utilization among seven hundred Hispanics in Los Angeles County revealed that while the prevalence of chronic ailments and disability was significant, 62% of those with activity limitation relied primarily on assistance from family members (Lopez-Aqueres et al., 1984). Investigation of service utilization among Korean elders in Los Angeles County found that while they were disadvantaged relative to non-Hispanic whites in activity limitation and chronic disease, utilization of community-based health and social services was significantly lower than for non-Hispanic whites. For the majority of the services less than 1% of older Koreans reported utilizing services, with two exceptions—9% reported utilizing transportation services and 10% reported that they had utilized the services of a senior center (Moon, Lubben, and Villa, 1995).

While low utilization of community-based services by minority elders is seen as reflecting their large supportive family networks and preferences for family support (Mindel and Wright, 1982), there is evidence that barriers exist that prevent utilization of services by older minorities (Damron-Rodriquez, Wallace, and Kington, 1994). Barriers to utilization include lack of knowledge about services, language problems, complex application processes, location of providers outside minority communities, and lack of bicultural staff (Moon, Lubben, and Villa, 1995; National Council of La Raza, 1991). The lack of culturally sensitive services is reported by African-American elders as a significant barrier to service use (Bailey, 1987; Jones-Morrison, 1986), and language barriers have been found to particularly impact use of services by Asian and Hispanic elders (Chee and Kane, 1983; Wallace, Levy-Storms, and Ferguson, 1995). Lack of awareness about the existence of services accounts for low participation rates among older Koreans. Specifically, when use was analyzed among older Koreans who knew about the services, utilization rates changed dramatically. Of those aware of the service, 18% used senior centers, 58% used transportation services, 50% sought advice about nutrition, 33% used visiting nurses, and 27% used the services of a home health aid (Moon, Lubben, and Villa, 1995). Clearly, these data demonstrate the need for legislation that mandates that providers create culturally appropriate and sensitive programs and develop outreach strategies targeted to minority communities.

Anti-Immigrant Legislation and Older Minorities

While anti-immigrant policies are not directed specifically at the elderly, seniors are nevertheless impacted and experience the effects of broader policy changes. An example from recent history is the passage of the Personal Responsibility and Work Opportunity Reconciliation Act referenced earlier in the chapter. While the intent of the legislation was to motivate able-bodied welfare recipients to work, it poses serious consequences for access to health care and income protection for elderly legal immigrants. Under the act legal immigrants will no longer be eligible for public assistance under SSI and therefore are ineligible for Medicaid. About one-fourth of SSI recipients are noncitizen legal immigrants (U.S. Social Security Administration, 1994). It is estimated that 500,000 legal immigrants will lose their benefits under SSI, 68% of whom are over age 65 and unable to work. The population considered most "at risk" are elderly legal immigrants reliant on Medicaid to cover the cost of nursing home stays and in-home supportive services. Additionally, the act makes immigrants ineligible for most federal benefits including welfare, unemployment benefits, food assistance, and public housing, and gives states the option to deny Medicaid to future legal immigrants (National Council of La Raza, 1996). While the most obvious effect of this legislation is that it will decrease access to basic health and social services to elderly immigrant populations, it also further feeds into and perpetuates anti-immigrant sentiments.

Anti-immigrant sentiment in the United States is reflected in public opinion polls and in support for anti-immigrant legislation. Moore (1993) found that 55% of Americans believe that immigrants cause economic crisis by increasing the demand for public services. Public support in California for Proposition 187, a law to make undocumented immigrants ineligible for all public services and to require service providers to identify undocumented users, and the recent attacks on affirmative action offer further evidence of negative sentiment toward immigrant populations. Anti-immigrant sentiment affects minority older persons by limiting their access to services: elders who have family members who are immigrants may be reluctant to use needed government services even when they are eligible because of fear of putting other family members at risk (Wallace and Villa, forthcoming). Moreover, the continued backlash toward immigrant populations is counterproductive to efforts aimed at designing policies and programs to improve the lives of older minorities.

Recommendations

The empirical evidence is clear; minority older persons are disproportionately disadvantaged for poor health and socioeconomic status and their families are experiencing vulnerabilities that impact their ability to care for older family members. It is also clear that in order to ensure that today's and tomorrow's generation of minority elders are not economically disadvantaged and physically vulnerable, we must pay attention to the issues of income security and health among younger generations of minority populations and find ways to support the family in caregiving activities. A recurring theme is that low educational attainment is related to low income, poverty, poor health, and social vulnerability. Therefore, educational opportunity is a primary point of intervention. Germane to any intervention in improving health and economic status, however, is the amelioration of social-structural barriers including racism, oppression, segregation, and antiminority sentiment—factors that preclude access to education, basic health, and opportunities for advancement, and, ultimately, limit life choices.

Improving Access to Health and Long-Term Care Services

Improving access to needed health and long-term care services among minority populations will require the adoption of some form of national health insurance that provides equal access to health care for all older Americans and provides nondiscriminatory cost control (Pepper Commission, 1990). Given the current climate of cost containment and program cutbacks, however, adoption of universal coverage will require a concentrated effort of broad coalitions of older and younger members of society joined together in advocacy (Wallace and Villa, forthcoming). Toward this end it is imperative that minority communities and organizations serving minority elders coalesce with mainstream aging organizations, groups representing children and other disadvantaged populations, as well as organized labor to advocate for policies that increase access and improve levels of care, and decrease barriers to utilization of health and long-term care services for all Americans. The fact that the number of uninsured individuals in the United States is approaching 44 million suggests that coalition building among these groups is long overdue.

Additionally, ensuring that health policy and long-term care programs are responsive to minority elderly populations will require minority-elected officials and national aging organizations representing minority populations to make health and long-term care a major part of their agendas and to develop proposals and platforms that are informed, visible, and well-suited for the populations they represent. The development of proposals for the financing, development, and delivery of health and long-term care will also require minority scholars and service providers to play a key role in educating policymakers about the needs and aging experience of minority elders. In addition, it is critical that communities, service providers, and advocacy groups work toward empowering older minorities to move toward self-advocacy by educating them about the policy process and about how public policy affects their lives. Educating policymakers and building a base of older minority populations that are informed advocates can ultimately lead to policy agendas that not only better serve their needs, but are more proactive (Wallace and Villa, forthcoming).

Improving Economic Security

In order to ensure a healthier more economically secure older minority population now and in the future, the issue of their income security must be addressed. One area of intervention is education. Specifically, resources must be invested to ensure that minority populations have the opportunity to acquire a decent and adequate education that will allow them to compete successfully for available employment opportunities. Many minority elderly populations are educationally disadvantaged (Gerontological Society of America, 1994). For example, over one-third of elderly Mexican-Americans and Hispanics have less than a fourth-grade education (Lacayo, 1993). This is clearly a disadvantage predictive of poverty, underemployment, and poor health across the life course. In order for future generations of minority elders to achieve economic well-being, given recent and proposed cutbacks in social welfare programs and in many forms of public assistance, it will become increasingly important to improve the options minority populations have for economic productivity through education, training, and job development (Morrison, 1990; Sheppard, 1990; Torres-Gil, 1992). A sign of hope for improving access to education for low-income and minority populations is found in recent proposals by President Clinton calling for increased funding for Head Start programs, expansion of the Pell grant for low-income students, tax breaks and savings incentives designed to make college more affordable for low-income populations, and the development of technology literacy programs that integrate computers into primary and secondary classrooms. Social policies that assist young people in completing high school, college, or vocational programs can reduce sporadic and low-paying employment that result in working conditions that can have a negative impact on health over the life course and can result in poor health in old age.

In addition, as a society we must increase efforts to eliminate racism and discrimination that block opportunities for education and employment, so important for improving socioeconomic and health status across the life course. Federally mandated programs that prohibit discrimination in employment and education should be passed and enforced (Malveaux, 1993). Meeting this goal will require moving beyond our current national mood of intolerance toward one that embraces diversity and that welcomes immigrant populations.

To improve economic security, attention must also be given to employment issues including the availability of job opportunities, job stability, and promotion for minority populations. Accordingly, phenomena such as "glass ceilings," occupational segregation, racial discrimination in employment, unequal pay for equal work practices, anti-immigrant sentiments and legislation—all which limit opportunity and advancement for minorities and women and therefore stunt economic stability—must be ameliorated (Chen, 1994). Likewise, as a society, we must address social barriers to economic stability including teen pregnancy, crime, violence, and drug abuse (Torres-Gil, 1992). These social problems disproportionately affect minority populations and have a negative impact on educational attainment, family stability, health, and economic stability across the life course. A lack of attention to these barriers now will mean the further perpetuation of an older minority population living in poverty and dependent on unstable, if not nonexistent, public programs.

Conclusion

These recommendations for policy intervention cannot and will not occur without attention to broader macroeconomic issues. Income security in old age or at any age is heavily dependent on, and influenced by, economic phenomena including growth, productivity, inflation, and unemployment (Chen, 1994). Recent cutbacks in federal programs, an economy that favors job creation in highly specialized areas, and the growth in low-paying service sector jobs suggest that without significant policy intervention future cohorts of minority elders will not be better off than the current cohort (Jackson, Lockery, and Juster, 1996; Stanford and Torres-Gil, 1991; Williams and Collins, 1995). Therefore, in considering ways to improve the health and economic status of minority populations we must examine the ways in which fiscal, monetary, and regulatory policies impact earnings, employment status, and savings across the life course. For example, the accumulation of national debt across the 1980s and early 1990s resulted in budget cuts to programs such as SSI that impact economic security among older persons (Chen, 1994). While individual efforts, employer-based retirement programs, pensions, and viable social insurance programs (i.e., Social Security) are all critical to economic security in old age, a productive and growing economy is the foundation of economic security and an area where increased attention among policymakers is long overdue (ibid.; see chapter by Chen in this volume).

Attention to these broader economic issues is often diverted by proposals such as the "Contract with America" and a political climate that calls for "individual responsibility." This kind of rhetoric is problematic not only because it erroneously assumes that there is equality of opportunity in the United States but because it also draws the public's attention away from the broader economic problems facing our society that are beyond individual control. Lack of growth in real wages, a dual labor market, inflation, stagflation, and erosion of pension income limit individual choice and opportunity. Until attention is paid to these issues, future cohorts of minority elders will continue to experience the vulnerabilities of their predecessors.

References

Administration on Aging (AOA). (1995). Medicaid block grants and OAA performance partnerships: Potential impacts on LTC for diverse communities. *Diversity and Long Term Care Newsletter.*

Advisory Council on Social Security. (1997). *Report of the 1994–1996 Advisory Council on Social Security.* Vol. I, Findings and Recommendations. U.S. Department of Health and Human Services: Washington, DC

Aleksa, K. (1994). *Income among Older Americans in 1992.* Washington, DC: American Association of Retired Persons.

American Association of Retired Persons (AARP). (1994). *A Profile of Older Americans.* Washington, D.C.: AARP Fulfillment.

Amott, T. L., and Matthaei, J. A. (1991). *Race, Gender, and Work: A Multicultural Economic History of Women in the United States.* Boston: South End Press.

Andersen, M. L. (1993). *Thinking about Women, 3rd ed.* New York: Macmillan.

Angel, J. L., and Hogan D. P. (1994). Demography of minority populations. In J. S. Jackson (Ed.), *Minority Elders Five Goals Toward Building a Public Policy Base. 2nd ed.*, pp. 9–21. Washington, DC: Gerontological Society of America.

Antonucci, T. C., and Cantor, M. H. (1994). Strengthening the family support system for older minority persons. In J. S. Jackson (Ed.), *Minority Elders Five Goals Toward Building a Public Policy Base. 2nd ed.*, pp. 40–45. Washington, DC: Gerontological Society of America.

Applewhite, S. R., and Daley, J. M. (1988). Cross-cultural understanding for social work practice with the Hispanic elderly. In S. R. Applewhite (Ed.), *Hispanic Elderly in Transition: Theory, Research, Policy, and Practice*, pp. 3–16. New York: Greenwood Press.

Bailey, E. J. (1987). Sociocultural factors and health care-seeking behavior among Black Americans. *Journal of the National Medical Association*, 79(4), 389–92.

Bayne-Smith, M. (1996). Health and women of color: A contextual overview. In M. Bayne-Smith (Ed.), *Race, Gender, and Health*, pp. 1–42. Thousand Oaks: Sage.

Becerra R. (1984). *The Hispanic Elderly*. New York: New York University Press.

Bradshaw, B., and Foner, E. (1978). The mortality of Spanish surnamed persons in Texas. In F. Bean and W. Frisbie (Eds.), *The Demography of Ethnic and Racial Groups*. New York: Academic.

Burton, L. M., Dilworth-Anderson, P., and Bengtson, V. L. (1991). Theoretical challenges for the Twenty-First Century: Creating culturally relevant ways of thinking about diversity and aging. *Generations*, fall/winter, 67–72.

Calasanti, T. M. (1996). Incorporating diversity: Meaning, levels of research, and implications for theory. *The Gerontologist*, 36(2), 147–56.

Cantor, M., and Mayer, M. (1976). Health and the inner-city elderly. *The Gerontologist*, 17, 17–24.

Center on Budget and Policy Priorities. (1989). Minimum wage veto hurts Latinos and Blacks. *Hispanic Link Weekly Report*, 26 June, pp. 2–4.

Chee, P., and Kane, R. (1983). Cultural factors affecting nursing home care for minorities: A study of Black American and Japanese American groups. *Journal of the American Geriatrics Society*, 31, 109–11.

Chen, Y. P. (1994). Improving the economic security of minority persons as they enter old age. In J. S. Jackson (Ed.), *Minority Elders Five Goals Toward Building a Public Policy Base, 2nd ed.*, pp. 22–31. Washington, DC: Gerontological Society of America.

Commonwealth Fund Commission Report. (1989). *Poverty and Poor Health among Elderly Hispanic Americans*. Baltimore: Commonwealth Fund Commission.

Damron-Rodriqueuz, J., Wallace, S., and Kington, R. (1994). Service utilization and minority elderly: Appropriateness, accessibility, and acceptability. *Gerontology and Geriatrics Education*, 15(1), 45–63.

Esping-Andersen, G. (1990). *The Three Worlds of Welfare Capitalism*. New Jersey: Princeton University Press.

Ferraro, K. F. (1987). Double jeopardy to health for Black older adults? *Journal of Gerontology*, 42, 528–33.

Garcia A. (1990). Social Security and the economic well-being of elderly minorities. In E. P. Stanford, F. Torres-Gil, and S. A. Schoenrock (Eds.), *Diversity in an Aging America: Challenges for the 1990s*, pp.16–26. San Diego: National Resource Center on Minority Aging Populations.

———. (1993). Income security and elderly Latinos. In M. Sotomayor and A. Garcia (Eds.), *Elderly Latinos: Issues and Solutions for the 21st Century*, pp. 17–28. Washington, DC: National Hispanic Council on Aging.

Gerontological Society of America (GSA). (1994). Introduction. In J. S. Jackson (Ed.), *Minority Elders: Five Goals Towards Building a Public Policy Base, Second Edition*, pp. 1–8. Washington, DC: GSA.

Gibson, R. C. (1991). The subjective retirement of Black Americans. *Journal of Gerontology: Social Sciences*, 46, S204–S209.

———. (1988). The work, retirement, and disability of older black Americans. In J. S. Jackson (Ed.), *The Black American Elderly: Research on Physical and Psychosocial Health*, pp. 304–24. New York: Springer.

Hanis C., Ferrell, R., Barton, S., Aguilar, L., Garza, A., Tulloch, B., Garcia, C., and W. Schull. (1983). Diabetes among Mexican Americans in Starr County, Texas. *American Journal of Epidemiology*, 118, 659–72.

Hyde, J. C., and Torres-Gil, F. M. (1991). Ethnic minority elders and the Older Americans Act: How have they fared? *Generations*, summer/fall, 57–61.

Jackson, J. J. (1988). Social determinants of the health of aging black populations in the United States. In J. J. Jackson (Ed.), *The Black*

American Elderly: Research on Physical and Psychosocial Health, pp. 69–98. New York: Springer.

Jackson, J., Lockery, S., and Juster, F. (1996). Introduction: Health and retirement among ethnic and racial minority groups. *The Gerontologist,* 36(3), 282–84.

John, R. (1990). The uninvited researcher in Indian country: Problems of process and product conducting research among Native Americans. *Mid-American Review of Sociology,* 14, 113–33.

———. (1994). The state of research on American Indian elders health, income security, and social support networks. In J. S. Jackson (Ed.), *Minority Elders: Five Goals Toward Building a Public Policy Base,* pp. 46–58. Washington, DC: GSA.

Johnson, R. J., and Wolinsky, F. D. (1994). Gender, race, and health: The structure of health status among older adults. *The Gerontologist,* 34(1), 24–35.

Jones-Morrison, B. (1986). The risk and access of Black elderly to institutional and noninstitutional continuing care services. Geriatric Society of America. Paper presentation.

Kaplan, G. A., Haan, M. N., Syme, S. L., Minkler, M., and Windeby, M. (1987). Socioeconomic status and health. In R. W. Amler and H. B. Dull (Eds.), *Closing the Gap: The Burden of Unnecessary Illness,* pp. 125–29. New York: Oxford University Press.

Kingson, E., and Quadagno, J. (1995). Social Seurity: Marketing Radical Reform. *Generations,* 14(3), 43–49.

Kiyak H. A., and Hooyman, N. R. (1994). Minority and socioeconomic status: Impact on quality of life in aging. In R. P. Abeles, H. C. Gift, and M. G. Ory (Eds.), *Aging and Quality of Life,* pp. 295–315. New York: Springer Publishing.

Krause, N. M. (1987). Stress in racial differences in self-reported health among the elderly. *The Gerontologist,* 27, 72–76.

Kraus, N., and Wray, L.A. (1991). Psychosocial correlates of health and illness among minority elders. *Generations,* fall/winter, 25–30.

Lacayo, C. G. (1993). Hispanic elderly: Policy issues in long-term care. In C. Barresi and D. Stull (Eds.), *Ethnic Elderly and Long-Term Care,* pp. 223–34. New York: Springer Publishing.

Lopez-Aqueres, W., Kemp, B., Plopper, M., Stables, F., and Brummel-Smith. (1984). Health needs of the Hispanic elderly. *Journal of the American Geriatric Society,* 32(3), 191–97.

Malveaux, J. (1993). Race, poverty, and women's aging. In J. Allen and A. Pifer (Eds.), *Women on the Front lines: Meeting the Challenge of an Aging America*, pp. 167–90. Washington, DC: Urban Institute Press.

Markides, K., and Black, S. A. (1996). Race, ethnicity, and aging: The impact of inequality. In R. H. Binstock and L. K. George (Eds.), *Handbook of Aging and the Social Sciences, Fourth Edition*, pp. 153–70. San Diego: Academic.

———, Coreil, J., and Rogers, L. (1989). Aging and health among Southwestern Hispanics. In K. Markides (Ed.), *Aging and Health, Perspectives on Gender, Race, Ethnicity, and Class*, pp. 177–210. Newbury Park: Sage Publications.

Markides, K., and Lee, D. (1990). Predictions of well-being and functioning in older Mexican Americans and Anglos: An eight year follow-up. *Journal of Gerontology,Social Sciences Edition*, 45(1), 69–73.

Markides, K., and Martin, H. (1983). *Older Mexican Americans: A Study in an Urban Barrio*. Austin: University of Texas Press.

Markides, K., and Mindel, C. H. (1987). *Aging & Ethnicity*. Beverly Hills: Sage Publications.

Mindel, C. H., and Wright, R. (1982). The use of social participation of Black and White elderly. *Aging and Human Development*, 2, 172–88.

Moon, A., Lubben, J. L., and Villa, V. (1995). Awareness and Utilization of Community Long-term Care Services by Elderly Korean and Non-Hispanic White Americans. Gerontological Society of America, Los Angeles, CA. Paper presentation.

Moore, D. (1993). Americans feel threatened by new immigrants. *Gallup Poll Monthly*, 334, 2–17.

Morrison, M. (1990). Economic well-being and the aging of minority populations. In E. P. Stanford, F.Torres-Gil, and S. A. Schoenrock (Eds.), *Diversity in an Aging America: Challenges for the 1990s*, pp. 4–15. San Diego: National Resource Center on Minority Aging Populations.

Mui, A. C., and Burnette, D. (1994). Long-term care service use by frail elders: Is ethnicity a factor? *The Gerontologist*, 34(2), 190–98.

Mutchler, J. E. and Burr, J. A. (1991). Racial differences in health and health care service utilization in later life: The effect of socioeconomic status. *Journal of Health and Social Behavior*, 32, 342–56.

National Center for Health Statistics (NCHS). (1984). Health indicators for Hispanic, Black, and White Americans. *Vital and Health Statis-*

tics. Series 10, no.148, PHHS Pub. no. 84 1576. Public Health Service, Washington, DC: U.S. Government Printing Office.

———. (1995). *Health in the United States, 1994*. Hyattsville, MD: U.S. Public Health Service.

National Council of La Raza (NCLR). (1991). *On the Sidelines: Hispanic Elderly and the Continuum of Care*. Washington, DC: NCLR.

———. (NCLR). (1992). *State of Hispanic America 1991: An Overview*. February. Washington, DC: NCLR.

———. (1996). *Immigration and Welfare Reform Legislation: The Impact on Latinos*. Washington, DC: NCLR.

National Research Council (1989). *A Common Destiny: Blacks and American Society*. Washington, DC: National Academy Press.

Newquist, D. (1976). *Prescriptions for Neglect: Experiences of Older Blacks and Mexican Americans with the American Health Care System*. Los Angeles: Andrus Gerontology Center, University of Southern California.

O'Donnel, R. (1989). Functional disability among the Puerto Rican elderly. *Journal of Aging and Health*, 1(2), 244–64.

Pepper Commission. (1990). *A Call for Action*. U.S. Bipartisan Commission on Comprehensive Health Care. Washington, DC: U.S. Government Printing Office.

Perez-Stable, E. J., McMillan, M. M., and Harris, M. I. (1989). Self-reported diabetes in Mexican Americans: HHANES 1982–84. *American Journal of Public Health*, 79, 770–72.

Riley, P. (1995). *Long-Term Care: The Silent Target of the Federal and State Budget Debate*. Washngton, DC: National Academy on Aging.

Sheppard, H. (1990). Work and productivity. In E. P. Stanford, F. Torres-Gil, and S. A. Schoenrock (Eds.), *Diversity in an Aging America: Challenges for the 1990s*, pp. 27–39. San Diego: National Resource Center on Minority Aging Populations.

Sotomayor, M. (1993). The Latino elderly: A policy agenda. In M. Sotomayor and A. Garcia (Eds.), *Elderly Latinos: Issues and Solutions for the 21st Century*, pp.1–15. Washington, DC: National Hispanic Council on Aging.

Stable, E., McMillen, M., Harris, M., Juarez, R., Knowler, W., Stern, M., and Haynes, S. (1989). Self reported diabetes in Mexican Americans. *American Journal of Public Health*, 79(6), 770–72.

232 *Valentine M. Villa*

Stanford, E. P., Torres-Gil, F., and S. A. Schoenrock. (1990). *Diversity in an Aging American: Challenges for the 1990s.* San Diego: National Resource Center on Minority Aging Populations.

Stanford, E. P., and Torres-Gil, F. M. (1991). Diversity and beyond: A commentary. *Generations,* fall/winter, 5–7.

Stanford, E. P., and Yee, D. (1991). Gerontology and the relevance of diversity. *Generations,* fall/winter, 11–14.

Stern, M., and Gaskill, S. (1978). Secular trends in ischemic heart disease mortality from 1970 to 1976 in Spanish surnamed and other white individuals in Bexar County, Texas. *Circulation,* 58, 537–43.

———, Hazuda, H., Gardner, L., and Haffner, S. (1983). Does obesity explain excess prevalence of diabetes among Mexican Americans? *Diabetologia,* 24, 272–77.

Stoller, E. P., and Gibson, R. C. (1994). Different worlds in aging: Gender, race, and class. In E. P. Stoller and R. C. Gibson (Eds.), *Worlds of Difference: Inequality in the Aging Experience,* pp. xvii-xxviii. Thousand Oaks, CA: Pine Forge Press.

Taeuber, C. M. (1992). Sixty-five plus in America. *Current Population Reports: Special Studies (Series P–23, no. 178.)* Washington, DC: U.S. Government Printing Office.

Torres-Gil, F. (1992). *The New Aging, Politics and Change in America.* New York: Auburn House.

U.S. Bureau of the Census. (1990). Poverty in the United States: 1990. *Current Population Survey Reports,* Series P–60, no. 175, Table 3, 18–19. Washington, DC: U.S. Government Printing Office.

———. (1992). *Statistical Abstract of the United States, 1992, 12th ed.* Washington, DC: U.S. Department of Commerce.

U.S. Social Security Administration. (1994). *Aliens Who Receive SSI Payments.* Baltimore, MD: Office of Supplemental Security Income.

Villa, V. M., Lubben, J. L., and Moon, A. (1995). Korean elderly health status: assessing the impact of sociodemographic, disease, and social support determinants on self-rated health and functioning. GSA, Los Angeles, CA. Paper presentation.

Villers Foundation. (1987). *On the Other Side of Easy Street: Myths and Facts about the Economic of Old Age.* Washington DC: Villers Foundation.

Wallace, S., and Manuel-Barkin, C. (1995). *Older Immigrants in California: Health Care Needs and the Policy Context.* Los Angeles: UCLA Center for Health Policy Studies.

Wallace, S., Levy-Storms, L., and Ferguson, L. (1995). Access to paid in-home assistance among disabled elderly people: Do Latinos differ from non-Latino whites? *American Journal of Public Health*, 85(7), 970–75.

Wallace, S., and Villa, V. (forthcoming). Caught in hostile cross-fire: Public policy and minority elderly in the United States. In K. Markides and M. Miranda (Eds.), *Minorities, Aging, and Health*. Sage: Beverly Hills.

Waller, J. B. (1989). Challenges to the provision of health care to minority aged. First annual summer symposium: Geriatric Education Center of Michigan. Ann Arbor, MI. June. Paper presentation.

Wiener, J. (1996). Can medical long-term care expenditures for the elderly be reduced? *The Gerontologist* 36(6), 800–11.

Williams, D. R. (1990). Socioeconomic differentials in health: A review and redirection. *Social Psychology Quarterly*, 53, 81–99.

Williams, D., and Collins, C. (1995). Socioeconomic and racial differences in health: Patterns and explanations. *Annual Review of Sociology*, 21, 349–86.

Chapter 12   *Read if time permits*

Aging as a Female Phenomenon:
The Plight of Older Women

JANIE S. STECKENRIDER

Mrs. Zella Smith, 86, is a widow who lives alone. Although Mrs. Smith did not work after marriage, as a widow of an eligible worker she receives Social Security and because she meets the minimum income standards she also receives Supplemental Security Insurance (SSI). Her combined monthly income is $458 ($5,496 annually). Last year Mrs. Smith broke her hip and was in the hospital. Medicare paid her hospital bill but the $716 deductible was covered by Medicaid that also pays Mrs. Smith's Medicare Part B monthly premiums and copayments. Medicaid pays for her prescription drugs, her eyeglasses, and hearing aid as well. She receives a hot meal delivered to her home Monday through Friday by the local Meals on Wheels program. There is a suggested donation of $2 per day that Mrs. Smith cannot afford but the program does not turn away individuals if they cannot pay. She also receives $63 in Food Stamps per month. Because of complications from her broken hip and arthritis, Mrs. Smith has problems dressing, walking, and bathing so her daughter Florence, 62, stops by before and after work to help her mother. Besides personal care and hygiene, Florence also does her mother's grocery shopping, house cleaning, and bill paying. Florence took unpaid leave to care for her mother full-time when she came home from the hospital, but Florence knows she cannot afford to do that again plus her boss is getting angry at her frequent sick days (her only recourse when she has to take her mother to the doctor). Since they cannot afford to hire in-home health care, Florence and Mrs. Smith both worry that the day is nearing when Mrs. Smith will have to go into a nursing home. Medicaid will pay for a skilled nursing facility, but both see that as a last resort.

The plight of Mrs. Zella Smith and her daughter Florence illustrates the reality and burden of an aging America for many women. It is women who are on the front lines of aging (Allen and Pifer, 1993). First, women over age 65 outnumber men by almost two to three and comprise the majority of the elderly population. Second, it is women who are providing most of the unpaid care to the frail, disabled, or functionally limited elderly. Caregiving for the elderly primarily means middle-age and older women providing care to very old women. And third, older women are far more likely than older men to face economic disadvantage and social isolation in their later years. Although women are 59% of the elderly population, they comprise 74% of the elderly poor (Taeuber, 1993) and over 6 million elderly women have incomes below 150% of the poverty level (Allen, 1993). For many older women, their "golden years" mean living alone one step from poverty and one female caregiver from a nursing home.

Paradoxically, most age-related policies developed from a male perspective of aging and are directed toward experiences of the male life cycle. Social Security benefits are calculated on a thirty-five-year continuous wage history and provide a spouse benefit based on a traditional couple of a breadwinner-husband and homemaker-wife. Pensions are associated with higher paying jobs and businesses with a larger employee base that more typically describes the male career. Medicare primarily provides coverage for acute health conditions and little for prevention or long-term care. It is older men who are far more vulnerable to fatal acute conditions, especially heart disease, while older women are more likely to suffer from chronic health conditions (Barer, 1994). The assumption of elderly caregiving by wives, daughters, and daughters-in-law no doubt has impeded policies of paid family leave, widespread community home care, and higher wages and benefits for the paid caregiving industry. While age-related policies are gender-neutral in language, they lead to gender-specific consequences: aging policies and programs based on a male model are most often providing services to older women, without recognizing that their aging experiences are not the same as those of older men.

This chapter explores aging as a female phenomenon. First the current reality of elderly women is examined with a focus on their demographic characteristics and factors associated with economic disadvantage, especially poverty. The implications for older women of age-related, male-based models are discussed in the areas of retirement income, health care, and caregiving. From this perspective the current political climate of program cutbacks and elimination is important to the well-being of older women. Last, the chapter looks to the future of aging policy for older women and how the increased labor force participation and higher education of young females may or may not hold brighter prospects for their old age.

A Profile of Older Women

Demographic Characteristics

There are over 33 million people aged 65 and over in the United States and they represent 12.7% of the population or about one in every eight Americans. The 19.7 million women outnumber the 13.5 million older men and comprise 59% of the elderly (American Association of Retired Persons, 1995). The sex ratio of the number of men to 100 women decreases with age among the elderly. At ages 65 to 69, there are 81 males for every 100 females and the ratio decreases to only 39 men to every 100 women among those over age 85 (Barer, 1994).

For much of the twentieth Century, the decrease in the number of births was the primary reason for the increase in the percent of the aging population. Now the improved survival to the oldest-old ages, especially among women, is the most important factor in the growth of the elderly (Rosenwaike and Dolinsky, 1987). The most dramatic decrease in mortality has been among oldest-old females, primarily due to decreases in cardiovascular disease (Fingerhut, 1984). Life expectancy is 75.5 years with nearly a seven-year difference between women at 78.7 years and men at 72.0 years (Crispell, 1995). At age 65, the average white male can expect to live 15.4 years and the African-American male 13.4 years compared to the life expectancy at age 65 for white females of 19.2 years and 17.2 years for African-American females (American Association of Retired Persons, 1995). These gender differences in life expectancy result in a high rate of widowhood and living alone among older females. On the positive side, women's increased longevity can mean added years of good health but also just as often are added years of chronic health problems, increased disability, and dependency.

The oldest-old, those aged 85 and over, are the fastest-growing segment of the population. This age group increased five times from 1950 to 1990 and is expected to grow from 3 million in 1990 to 8 million in 2030 and then to 15 million in 2050. In 2010, one-fifth of elderly women are expected to be over the age of 85 (Taeuber, 1993). Today's oldest-old are comprised of about 850,000 men and 2.2 million women. The number of very old women is expected to increase to 5.6 million by 2030 and to 10 million by 2050 (ibid.). Although individuals over age 85 have better health than in previous decades and can expect remaining years of independent life, this age group overall has greater impairment, more social isolation, a higher need for social services, less income, and a heightened need for caregiving. Many problems and burdens of aging are actually those of the oldest-old and are overwhelmingly problems of females. This female-dominated age segment heavily utilizes age-related public policies and social programs, including Social Security, Medicare, Medicaid, transportation and meal programs, legal assistance, low-income energy assistance, and homemaker assistance.

A key gender difference with policy implications is marital status. Most elderly men (77%) are married while most elderly women are not (41%) with even greater differences over age 75, 70% of men are married compared to 25% of females. In fact, elderly women are three times more likely than elderly men to be widowed (49% of females, 14% of males). Approximately 5% of the elderly are divorced and have not remarried (Saluter, 1991). Given females' longer life expectancy and the pattern of women marrying men a few years older, the rate of widowhood among older women increases with age. About one third of women are widowed by age 65, over one-half by age 75, and 80% of women are widowed by age 80 (Holden, 1989). Though the joint survival of couples has increased and the age of widowhood has been postponed, today's 65-year-old woman can expect to live nearly 15 years past the death of her spouse (ibid.).

The differences in marital status of older males and females have important effects. Because of the high rate of widowhood, older women are more likely than older men to live alone. In 1990, there were 9.2 million persons over age 65 living alone and 78.8% of them were female (Saluter, 1991). The condition of living alone is one factor highly associated with poverty among the elderly (see Taeuber, 1993; Malveaux, 1993; Allen, 1993). Of seniors living alone, 23% were poor while only 6% of older persons living in families were poor (American Association of Retired Persons, 1995). Once widowed, women have fewer sources of income and receive lower Social Security benefits than when they were married. In fact, according to Estes, three-fourths of poor elderly females were not poor prior to the death of their spouse (Kleyman, 1995). Another consequence of the gender differences in marriage is caregiving support. Since most older men are married, they have a spouse to care for them if they suffer from poor health or limitation in activities of daily living. To illustrate, among those over age 85 who are functionally dependent 36% of the males live with a spouse compared to only 4% of the females and 38% of the functionally dependent women aged 65 to 84 live alone (Hing and Bloom, 1990). Because older women are likely to be unmarried and living alone, they are dependent on family, friends, and public programs for caregiving needs. It is no surprise therefore that women are far more likely than men to end up in a nursing home where three-fourths of the residents over age 65 are female (Taeuber, 1993).

Poverty

During the last thirty years, there has been a dramatic decline in the overall poverty rate of the elderly. In 1959, 35% of the elderly were considered poor compared to 12% in 1990. But important subgroup differences continue and the elderly poor are disproportionately female, ethnic, and live alone (Littman, 1991; Malveaux, 1993; American Association of Retired Persons, 1995). The 15.5% poverty rate for older women is twice that of older men (7.9%) and increases to 20% for women over age 75 (10% for males over age 75) (Taeuber, 1993; Braus, 1992). Even though the poverty rate for older women is lower than among children under age 18, the rate is higher than exists for females of other ages and it is very old females who are the most vulnerable (Malveaux, 1993). Poverty among the elderly strongly relates to marital status, living arrangement, and education. Elderly persons not living with relatives (living alone or with unrelated persons) are more likely to be poor (24.7%) than are elderly married couples (5%) (Taeuber, 1993). Put another way, about one-fourth of elderly females who live alone are poor and three-fourths of those in poverty, live alone (Malveaux, 1993). The higher rate of poverty among elderly female widows than among married couples is partly explained by the decreased income following the death of the spouse and because widows as a group are older than married females, have lower Social Security benefits from lower wages, and are less likely to receive a pension

(Holden, 1989). Hurd (1990) estimates that there is a 30% average increase in poverty after widowhood because of the permanent change in economic resources. Economic status among the elderly, as over the lifespan, is related to education and poverty decreases as the elderly's educational level increases (Taeuber, 1993). This relationship between economic status and education may be an important factor for the future of elderly women since a greater portion of Baby Boomer females have completed high school and college than have today's elderly females (ibid.).

Although bleak, the poverty data underestimate the reality of the economic situation of older women, many for whom poverty is just an accident waiting to happen. The majority of elderly women are not poor, but the average elderly female lives within poverty's reach. Fifteen percent of elderly females who are poor and one-third of older women who are near-poor have an income within 150% of the poverty line (Malveaux, 1993). This proportion of near-poor older females living between 100% and 150% of the poverty line is higher than among females aged 25 to 64 (Littman, 1991). The average median income for older women is only 28% above the poverty line (U.S. Bureau of the Census, 1991) and just 55.2% of all elderly women are considered "out of the woods" with an income at least two times the poverty level (Malveaux, 1993). Many of the elderly women not in poverty or near-poor are still married and may later suffer diminished income when widowed.

The poverty and near poverty of elderly women is a logical outcome of their set of work, retirement, health care and family norms, and public policies. Elderly women's economic status reflects their past experiences of years as nonpaid homemakers, jobs with low pay, occupational segregation during their working years, and responsibilities for child and elder care. The notion of the three-legged stool of financial resources in old age (Social Security, savings, and pensions) has been unattainable. Poor and near-poor women (and their spouses) are more likely to have been in relatively lower-paying jobs that made it difficult to accumulate savings. Now they receive lower Social Security benefits based on their (or their spouse's) lower wages and are unlikely to receive a pension (only 22% of women over 65 received a pension income in 1992) (Rothstein, 1994). These poor and near-poor women are more reliant on Social Security for income than the nonpoor. The average poor elderly person receives 80% of her total income from Social Security (Malveaux, 1993). For about one-third of unmarried elderly women, Social Security provides 90% of their income (Muller,

1983) and for 60% of elderly women Social Security is the sole income source (Older Women's League, 1991).

For the poor and near-poor elderly female, governmental programs for health care, transportation, Food Stamps, and homemaker assistance provide a supporting leg for her financial stool. The services provided by federal and state programs help lessen the consequences of limited economic resources. For many elderly, governmental social spending makes the difference, as Taylor (1991) estimates that 86% of the elderly who would be poor are lifted out of poverty by government tax and transfer programs. Government programs like SSI, a joint federal and state effort, guarantee a minimum income to those meeting the low-income and asset standards. About 10% of the elderly receive SSI and 75% of the recipients are female (U.S. Department of Health and Human Services, 1990).

Even the best financially prepared woman may be unable to protect herself from poverty in her later years. An unexpected ill husband can drain a couple's assets from the high cost of long- term care, the continuing need and expense of home health care, or the need to "spend down" to qualify for Medicaid coverage. Moreover, because the economic status of older women reflects their past experiences, it is difficult to address elderly poverty through social policy targeted strictly to the elderly (Malveaux, 1993). Earlier interventions into the female economic life span are necessary such as better and equal pay, discouraging gender discrimination in hiring, benefits for part-time workers, and increased pension portability.

This profile of elderly women highlights how aging is a woman's issue because of the skewed sex ratio, longer life expectancy, and greater need for services. The gender patterns of these demographic characteristics demonstrate that the aging experience is not the same for males and females. The prospect for a good old age is worse for women on every dimension including chronic health conditions, living alone, widowhood, poverty, and lack of economic resources. This confluence of demographics of the aging and gender intersects with the political climate of retrenchment. As this profile points out, policymakers' increased questioning of the elderly's disproportionate consumption of resources falls most heavily on older women. Reductions in government benefits and cutbacks in age-related public programs have their greatest impact and consequences on the lives of the most vulnerable who are overwhelmingly elderly females. For many older women, like Mrs. Zella Smith profiled at the beginning of this chapter, even small changes in the safety net of governmental programs can mean choices between basic items such as rent, food, medical care, prescriptions, or home heating.

Aging Policies from a Male Model

Despite the fact that the majority of older persons are female, that most Social Security beneficiaries are female, and that the bulk of elder care is females giving care to very old females, aging public policies have been shaped by assumptions based on the male life experience. Although age related public policies, past and present, have not developed with the intent of deliberate gender bias, the male life cycle has been the standard for policy decisions. Gender differences, outlined in the previous profile, and the policy assumptions of the male life cycle have led to gender specific effects from aging programs. Hess (1985) noted that the aging debate has been framed in masculine terms while the real problems of the elderly are disproportionately experienced by women and that females will increasingly bear the brunt of dealing with their consequences.

Retirement Income: Social Security

The primary economic support in retirement is Social Security and over nine out of ten older persons receive benefits from this safety net (O'Grady-LeShane, 1990). The foundations of this program based on worker productivity are closely tied to the patterns of the male life cycle and work to the disadvantage of women (Hudson, 1996). Gender biases in the program outcomes stem from benefit levels based on wages, use of a 35-year work history for benefits calculation, assumption of a breadwinner and homemaker couple, penalties to a dual earner family, and partial benefits for divorced spouses. An older woman in a couple is advantaged by the program's assumptions, but often finds herself with substantially less income when she outlives her husband.

Social Security is a wage-based program—benefit levels are tied to wages. This structure continues the relative economic status of men and women from the younger years into older age. Individuals in jobs with low wages, subsequently pay less into Social Security and then receive less in monthly benefits than persons in higher-paying jobs. Although many of the current female beneficiaries were not employed, the work history of retired working women tends to be in low-paying jobs. Females' lower earnings then continue into old age with lower Social Security benefits. The average monthly benefit of retired female workers is 76% of males (O'Grady-LeShane, 1990; Rayman, Allshouse, and Allen, 1993) and this ratio would be even lower if Social Security was not weighted toward higher replacement to low-income workers.

Gender bias results from the calculation of Social Security benefits based on a 35-year work history. To determine the benefit amount, the worker's contributions are averaged over 35 years with a zero included for each year out of the work force. This calculation method assumes the male pattern of continuous work history and penalizes the employment norm of women who tend to enter and leave the labor force for caregiving responsibilities. Only 12% of females over age 62 in 2010 will have spent 35 years in the labor force and only 22% of the youngest retired women, ages 62 to 69, would meet the standard (Zedlewski et al., 1990). Even in 2030 when the current generation of younger women retire, women who as a group have spent more years in the labor force than earlier female cohorts, only one-third will have worked continuously for 35 years. The remaining two-thirds will have zeros averaged into their benefits calculation (Fierst and Campbell, 1988). Even though an individual can drop five zeros, this allowance does not compensate for gender differences in work history. Women average 11.5 years out of the labor force while males average only 1.3 years (Leonard and Loeb, 1992).

In 1935 when Social Security began, the traditional division of labor within the family of a working husband and a homemaker-wife was incorporated into the program. Since that time, there have been decreased births, increased divorce, and increased female labor force participation that have eroded the traditional arrangements of the benefit structure (Gilbert, 1994). Less than 10% of families today fit the traditional family model of Social Security (Leonard and Loeb, 1992) but the assumptions remain and continue to privilege those who are married. Again, the incongruence between the program assumptions and realities are more onerous for women. As the demographic profile indicates, elderly men tend to be married and elderly women are likely to be single (widowed) and live alone.

Since 1939, Social Security has provided families the protection of a safety net in the form of dependent benefits for the spouse while the worker is alive and continued spousal benefits after the worker's death. Aimed at providing an adequate income for a couple, assuming a male worker and female homemaker, Social Security provides dependent benefits to the spouse that are 50% of the retired worker's benefit and later provides 100% of the worker spouse's benefit as widow protection on his death. However, if the wife has contributed to Social Security from her own employment, she is considered dually entitled and can qualify for either dependent benefits or benefits based on her own employment, whichever is higher. If she chooses benefits based on her own contributions, there are no changes in the amount nor is there widow protection after her husband's death. Therefore, the widow who previously received dependent benefits is now receiving two-thirds of the couple's income (the couple's income was 150% of the worker's benefit comprised of 100% worker's benefits and 50% dependent's benefits and later as a widow receives 100% of the worker's benefits). But the widow receiving benefits on her own contributions may be forced to live on only 50% of the couple's previous income if both were contributing equally (the couple's income was 50% from the husband and 50% from the wife and later the widow continues to receive only her 50%). Dual entitlement on its face is not biased against women but the reality for most retired females is lower benefits from their own worker contributions and higher benefits with greater long-term economic gains as a dependent.

Given the inequities in the system and the employment history of women concentrated in low-paying jobs, most women receive dependent benefits based on their husband's contributions. The percentage of women drawing Social Security as dependents has remained constant at 62% since 1962 although the percentage of women dually entitled has increased 22% (Leonard and Loeb, 1992). With the assumptions of traditional gender roles and family structure plus the low wages of women, Social Security advantages married couples and penalizes two-earner couples so many receive lower benefits than a one-worker couple.

Divorced women are also disadvantaged by Social Security. A divorced individual married less than ten years does not qualify for dependent spouse benefits. However, a longer marriage does entitle the individual to dependent spouse benefits. Like the dependent benefits for a married couple, the divorced wife receives a benefit equal to 50% of her worker husband's benefits or, if dually entitled, she can receive benefits based on her own worker contributions. The bias toward marriage is evident since the married couple receives three times the income (150% of the worker benefits) than the divorced wife who receives only 50% of the ex-spouse's benefits amount. Often the divorced older woman is left with an inadequate income that is not enough to live on. This Social Security rule may be increasingly important and affect more older women as the percentage of divorced, not remarried, females over age 65 is projected to increase from 5% in 1990 to 14% in 2020 (Taeuber, 1993).

Retirement Income: Pensions

One of the legs of the three-legged stool of retirement income is pensions. In 1940 pensions were rare with only 15% of all private and salary workers covered, but have become increasingly available (Turner and Beller, 1989). Pension coverage has accelerated and by 1988, 46% of private sector employees and 83% of public sector employees were covered by a pension (Hurd, 1990). This improved pension coverage has not translated into gender parity, however, since twice as many men over age 65 (46%) receive a pension compared to the percentage of older women (23.5%) (Leonard and Loeb, 1992). Women with a pension also receive less in benefits than males. In 1993, the average combined Social Security and pension income for males was $1,160 a month, 45% higher than the mean of $800 for women (Taeuber, 1993). Part of this difference is because female retirees are older and had lower relative earnings in earlier decades, but at each age group men have a higher pension income (Short and Nelson, 1991). Like Social Security, pensions are structured on the male employment pattern and while not gender biased on the surface, pensions disadvantage women in coverage and benefits.

Women's work patterns of entering and leaving the work force for caregiving, employment in low paying jobs, overrepresentation in part-time work, and concentration in jobs in small businesses reduce or deny them pension coverage. Pensions are structured on a continuous work history with most pension programs requiring five years to be vested. This tilts pensions toward the male job history as the median job tenure for males is 5.1 years and 3.7 years for females (Malveaux, 1993). For example, if a male and female both worked continuously for forty years, he in one job and she in four different jobs with the same pension plan, his pension would be twice hers (Leonard and Loeb, 1992). Women are penalized by their higher job mobility and shorter job tenure as they switch jobs or leave the work force because of family responsibilities, to escape a dead end job, or for caregiving. Males at all ages have higher pension coverage and vesting rates than female workers. In 1987, 64% of female workers had pension coverage and 40%

were vested compared to 69% of males with pension coverage and 49% vested (Malveaux, 1993).

Women are also disadvantaged by the pension system because of where they work. Women are overrepresented in part-time work, small businesses, and low-paying jobs that are not associated with pension coverage. Females are two-thirds of all part-time workers (Rayman et al., 1993) and 26% of all female workers are employed part-time (Callaghan and Hartmann, 1991). Among employers with less than 25 employees, 25% have a pension plan versus 89% of employers with over 1,000 employees (Leonard and Loeb, 1992). Concentration in low-paying jobs also decreases women's likelihood of pension coverage. Less than one-half of workers who earn less than $1,000 a month are in a pension plan while three-fourths of those earning more have pension coverage (ibid.). Without mandatory coverage and portability for pensions, these different factors of women's work patterns are obstacles in their pension coverage.

Women's longer life expectancy and greater likelihood of outliving their husbands also disadvantage them in the pension system. At his death, the husband's pension, which may have comprised a considerable portion of the couple's income, generally stops. The loss of this economic resource is a contributor to the 30% average increase in poverty after widowhood (Hurd, 1990). Only 3% of widows receive a surviving spouse pension because most couples waive the survivor benefits for higher benefits when both are alive (Leonard and Loeb, 1992).

Health Care

Medicare is the primary public program that provides health care coverage for older women. Modeled after the private insurance industry, Medicare is geared toward acute care and provides for hospital visits and doctor services. This health care coverage is more aligned with the needs of older men who are prone to accidents, heart disease, and "killer" conditions (Leader, 1988; Hess, 1985). Older men are more likely to suffer acute conditions that end in death while older women generally suffer from chronic conditions resulting in disability (Zones et al., 1987). Medicare is structured to deal with acute conditions and their treatment. It covers the costs of surgery, X rays, lab tests, radiation, diagnostic testing, inpatient hospital care, and inpatient care at a skilled nursing facility following a hospital stay (which means after an acute condition). Medicare tends not to cover those expenses associated with managing chronic conditions such as prescription or over-the-counter medications, hearing aids, glasses, routine foot care, or long-term care in a nursing home. Hess (1985) suggests that the types of health services likely to be needed by older women are out-of-pocket expenses.

Although most elderly females have Medicare, they still spend a significant portion of their income on health care. While Medicare's coverage was not created with gender specific intentions, the longer life expectancy of women and their ensuing health care needs have resulted in older women's higher out-of-pocket expenses compared to older men. Unmarried females over age 65 (primarily widows) spend an average of 16% of their income on health care compared to 9% for elderly married couples (Lamphere-Thorpe and Blendon, 1993). Medicare paid 49% of the health care expenses of elderly unmarried males in 1986 but only 33% for elderly females (Older Women's League, 1989).

Medicare's lack of coverage for most preventative health care services parallels the overall low priority of health prevention since only 3.4% of the country's total health care budget is directed toward this purpose (Fahs, 1993). A routine physical examination and related tests are not covered by Medicare nor are most immunizations. Mammograms, the most effective means to detect breast cancer, are a recent addition to Medicare coverage but the large copayment is often too high for low- and middle-income women (Kleyman, 1995). Despite the fact that half of all new cases of breast cancer are women aged 65 and older, two out of three older females do not get regular mammograms (U.S. Department of Health and Human Services, 1995). In short, Medicare's focus on acute care and technology does not protect women from preventable health problems. In 1994, only 44% of elderly women had a mammogram, 39% had a complete physical examination, 36% had a pelvic exam, 33% had a clinical breast exam, and 11% had a blood pressure check (Kleyman, 1995). The rates for preventative care are even lower for minority older women.

While the belief in health care has been that the long-term savings of prevention do not outweigh the costs, Fahs (1993) suggests that preventative care for elderly females will save both money and years of life. She sees prevention as cost-effective, especially for high risk older women, and necessary to avoid the high rate of disability and future health care costs. Perry and Butler (1988) predict that if medicine could delay the beginning of the decline from diseases of aging by just five years, the number with chronic disease and expenditures would be decreased by at least one-half. Lamphere-Thorpe and Blendon (1993) also point to the savings from the prevention of disability that can delay the need for costly long-term care.

While Medicare concentrates on acute care and hospital stays, elderly women are faced with a major gap in their health care coverage from inadequate long-term care financing. Given the demographic trends previously discussed of elderly women likely to be unmarried, live alone, be very old, and have chronic conditions, they disproportionately comprise the residents of nursing homes. Three-fourths of the residents in skilled nursing facilities are female (Taeuber, 1993; Lamphere-Thorpe and Blendon, 1993) and elderly women are twice as likely as older men to be in a nursing home (Hess, 1985). Since Medicare does not reimburse nursing home costs (except after a hospital stay for an acute condition), older women either have to pay out-of-pocket or meet the income means test for Medicaid. Depending on a state's minimum income level, poor older women may qualify for Medicaid that will cover long-term care. Older women above the state's means test often have no choice but to "spend down" their assets in order to qualify for Medicaid's coverage.

Medicaid is a vital provider of health care services to older women beyond Medicare so any reforms and reductions in the program are issues on the women's policy agenda. For older women who qualify, Medicaid not only provides long-term care but also covers Medicare's premiums and deductibles plus basic health care needs, including prescription drugs, eyeglasses, hearing aids, and medical equipment.

Caregiving

As the percentage and number of elderly have increased, especially the very old and frail elderly, the need for caregiving has also grown. The increased need for elder care is borne by females with many struggling to balance their dual roles of caregiver and worker. Caregiving is a women's issue because it is disproportionately women providing the care, both paid and unpaid, and it is mostly older women receiving the care. Elder care is a low priority on the public agenda and is facing diminished resources, yet society assumes and depends on women to provide the $700 billion to $1.4 trillion in unpaid care each year (Prescod, 1991).

There is no historical precedent for the coming experience of most middle-age and young-old persons having living parents (see chapter by Parrott in this volume). The parent support ratio, the number of persons over age 85 to every 100 persons aged 50–64 has increased threefold from 3 in 1950 to 9 in 1990. This ratio is expected to more than triple again by 2050 to 28 (Taeuber, 1993). With lowered mortality and improved survival at older ages, there is a heightened incidence of chronic conditions and the need for help. Among those over age 85, one-fifth have a problem with a major activity and two-fifths suffer from a condition that limits their activities (Taeuber, 1993). A 1990 study found 4.4 million elderly needing help with one or more ADLs (activity of daily living) (Harpine, McNeil, and Lamas, 1990).

Caregiving for the elderly parallels traditional notions about gender and family responsibility and presumes the unpaid labor of female relatives. Women—wives, daughters, daughters-in-law, granddaughters and nieces—provide the bulk of care to elderly relatives. Sons and husbands are relatively absent from caregiving (Aronson, 1992) with one study finding that men comprise only 21% of caregivers (Select Committee on Aging, 1988). There are also gender differences in the division of labor in caregiving that parallel traditional gender roles. While women assist the elderly in high intensity personal care tasks such as bathing, feeding, and toileting, men provide help with financial duties of bill paying, banking, and asset management (Foster and Brizius, 1993). Males are also far less likely to take time off from work for caregiving responsibilities (Leonard and Loeb, 1992).

About 80% to 90% of elder care is informally provided by the family. The average caregiver is a 57-year-old female but 36% of caregivers are over age 65 (Select Committee on Aging, 1988). The majority of caregivers provide assistance for one to four years and 20% for over five years. Eighty percent report giving care seven days a week (Stone, Cafferata, and Sangl, 1987). A study of female caregivers for family members over age 70 found that caregivers averaged 12 hours a week for personal care and 26 hours of care for the home—most while employed full-time (Gibeau, 1989). If the elderly relative lived with the caregiver, the combined individual and home care was 35 hours a week. Caregiving assistance includes such tasks as household chores, buying medications, transportation, shopping, changing bandages, managing finances, and personal care. Two-thirds of caregivers help with personal needs of

dressing, eating, toileting, and about one-half help with transferring in and out of bed (Foster and Brizius, 1993). Caregiving can
take a physical toll as well as mean less time for oneself, decreased
social life, and role conflict.

The growth in the elderly population and the greater need for
caregiving have coincided with the increased participation of women
in the labor force. In 1991, 57% of women over age 16 were employed and the highest rate was among women age 25 to 54 (74%).
Women's labor force participation is expected to increase 20% over
the next thirty years (Taeuber, 1993). The two trends of the increased demand for elder care and the greater employment of women
collide and result in role conflict for many women. Women in these
dual roles are often faced with difficult choices of missing time
from work, lower job productivity, taking a part-time job, or quit-
ting their job. Gibeau's study (1989) found that most women were
employed before becoming a caregiver and the majority have been
in the labor force for more than twenty years. The role conflict from
caregiving and a job creates worker stress, decreased productivity,
lateness, unscheduled absences, excessive use of the telephone, and
high absenteeism (Barr, Johnson, and Warshaw, 1992). Over 50%
of caregivers report having missed work during the last seven years
because of caregiving responsibilities (Gibeau, 1989).

The strain of caregiving coupled with job responsibilities can
ultimately mean that a woman leaves the labor force or finds a
part-time job for greater flexibility. Stone, Cafferata, and Sangl
(1987) found that 12% of females caring for their elderly parents
quit their job and a study by Brody (1987) of caregiving daughters
found that 13% left their jobs to take care of their elderly mothers.
A caregiver's decision to quit her job has consequences beyond lost
salary. It also means giving up employer-provided health care insurance, pensions, and contributions to Social Security. For a middle-
aged and older woman, giving up a job for caregiving comes at the
time when she needs to prepare for her own retirement. Social
Security, for example, does not recognize her years of unpaid
caregiving and averages zeros into the calculation of her benefits
level. The choice of part-time employment may help in the short-
run to continue earnings, but because part-time jobs rarely have
benefits she is disadvantaged in the long-run in terms of her own
retirement income.

Public policies to assist female caregivers in maintaining their
elderly relatives in the community are few. Aronson (1992) sees
elder care relying heavily on the taken for granted notion that this

is naturally a family responsibility (and ultimately a female responsibility). Public health and social services provide only 10% to 15% of total elder care (ibid.) with the rest assumed by the family. Community care has been poorly funded and continues to be a low priority on the policy agenda (in part because of the reliance upon unpaid female caregivers). There are minimal public moneys for home services such as homemaker assistance to shop or clean; the personal care of bathing, dressing, or feeding; and delivered meals.

Medicare does provide some home health care but the type of care provided by most female caregivers is not covered. Intermittent nursing care is paid by Medicare but this consists of generally brief visits from a nurse to change bandages, to administer injections, or to check blood pressure. The routine activities for daily living of food preparation, toileting, bathing, dressing, or transferring out of bed are not provided by Medicare. These are out-of-pocket expenses and are not reimbursed. With the structure of Medicare and Medicaid, it costs the elderly less to be in the hospital than to remain at home.

It is elderly widows and their female caregivers who are primarily affected by the public policies of caregiving and the lack of available and affordable community care. An older male is likely to be married and to have a caregiver-wife if he requires help with any ADLs. Older women, likely to be widowed and living alone, are dependent on others for care and it is their female relatives who assist them. Public policies are directed away from community care and the few public moneys available for this purpose are being further cut. One can only speculate what the caregiving system would be like if life expectancies were reversed and if a large proportion of older men could expect to end their lives alone in need of assistance for routine daily activities. The current caregiving system where males are basically nonexistent relies on women to provide the care needed by the elderly (mostly by females) at the same time that the economic system and public policies penalize women for their caregiving activities.

Future Prospects and Changes

The current political climate of program reductions and cutbacks reflects a general movement in government toward divestment. The theme in recent years has been to reduce the role of the federal government in providing income, health care, housing, transportation, and social services to the elderly. The multiple cuts in benefits and services have piled up and threaten the elderly's safety net. The program reductions have also been accompanied by a movement toward the elderly assuming more of the costs. For example, the growth in Medicare and health services have been scaled back at the same time Medicare's premiums have increased.

Any reduction in Social Security, Medicare, Medicaid, the Older Americans Act, or Food Stamps is inherently an issue on the women's agenda. It is women who are most vulnerable—as beneficiaries of programs providing fewer services and as caregivers who will need to provide even more care in the absence of public support. This interrelationship of government programs, cutbacks, and consequences for females is evident in the recent shift in Medicare. Medicare has decreased the average length of hospital stays at the same time that governmental support for home care has diminished. One consequence is a heightened need for female caregivers who provide the necessary care for the elderly person who lives alone to leave the hospital and return home. In all, the consequences of the reductions in old-age programs are increased out-of-pocket expenses for an elderly population that is predominantly female, unmarried, living alone, and with few economic resources.

Each of the three areas of retirement income, health care, and caregiving can achieve greater gender justice with new approaches to public policies. Even if the idea of gender justice in public support is not a high priority on the government agenda in the political environment of cutbacks (Aronson, 1992), an examination of possible changes is instructive. To achieve gender balance in programs would require marginal change in some public policies and massive overhaul in others, which is unlikely to occur. Yet these proposed changes, even if nonviable, can provide the foundation for future political debates.

Retirement income from both Social Security and pensions needs to be changed so that they do not continue the inequities for elderly females. Reforms are needed for the system to more fairly and accurately reflect the life patterns and retirement needs of the mostly female elderly. One change is dependent care credits that could be instituted to provide benefit credits for the years a worker was out of the labor force providing care to children or to elderly relatives without income covered by Social Security. An alternative in the calculation for Social Security benefits would be to drop out the years when the individual was providing family care and eliminate the zeros averaged into the benefits base. Similarly, a 25-year earnings history instead of the current 35-year standard could be used for benefits calculations and would better reflect the work history of women.

The worker/dependent structure of Social Security could be done away with for an earnings sharing system where a married couple would pool their earned Social Security contributions and split them at retirement, divorce, death, or disability. Although this totally revamps the system, the sharing of Social Security would recognize the contribution of women's unpaid caregiving years to the family structure. Less dramatic but also spurring a movement away from dependent benefits would be benefit equality for widows. A widow who receives benefits on her own worker contributions should receive two-thirds of the couple's previous benefits as now occurs for a widow receiving dependent benefits. Furthermore, an optional increased widow's benefit could be implemented that would allow the retired worker to voluntarily accept lower benefits in return for higher benefits to the surviving spouse. This would be one way to provide a better income for longer-living females.

Private pensions also need to be more in line with women's labor force participation. The length of job tenure for vesting and the lack of portability decrease the likelihood that women will receive a pension. Mandatory changes in these two areas to fewer vesting years and required portability would better mirror the shorter job tenure of women and ensure them a pension. Reforms to widen pension eligibility to part-time workers and to improve incentives for small businesses to provide a pension would also increase pension availability to women since they tend to be concentrated in these type of jobs.

However, as changes in Social Security and pensions are necessary for greater gender equity, without fundamental changes in the economic system women will continue to be disadvantaged in their old age. If women remain segregated in low-paying jobs with few benefits and fewer opportunities, they will still be unprotected in their later years. Pay equity and equal pay policies need to be a priority to raise the economic position of younger, employed women. Discrimination in hiring, training, education, and promotions must be eliminated so that women can be more competitive in the labor force. Improving job opportunities and benefits for female workers will improve their prospects in retirement.

Elderly health care portends to be one of the most explosive and accessible targets for program cutbacks especially since one-third of the nation's health care budget is consumed by the elderly.

The government shutdowns over the 1995 federal budget demonstrated the importance of elderly health care financing. Universal health care would improve the health condition of younger persons giving them increased access to medical services and treatment so that they would enter old age in better health. However, the failure of the Clinton administration's proposed health care plan shows once again, that national health insurance may be an American pipe dream. Any governmental reform in health care will be marginal at most and in large part dictated by the private health care and insurance industries.

Therefore, narrower goals will have to be pursued in health care reform. An increased targeting of preventive care for elderly women could have wide-ranging consequences. Given women's longer life expectancy, greater disability, and higher poverty level, increased preventative care and reimbursement for such services would mean significant economic savings. Medicare currently provides little in preventative care (i.e., vaccines for pneumococcal pneumonia and hepatitis B, mammograms, and Pap smears), but pays much more in the long run for the higher expenses of not initially preventing conditions. More attention to prevention would advantage both Medicare by arresting health conditions in earlier treatable stages and in older women who could gain improved morbidity.

Two currently debated reforms in health care, medical vouchers and turning Medicaid into a block grant, would have negative outcomes for elderly females. A medical voucher would be given to the Medicare beneficiary who would shop for her health care. This would put elderly persons, most who are female, at risk by requiring them to go into the health care market, be price sensitive, and to demand responsible care. Carroll Estes, former president of the Gerontological Society of America, sees this as unrealistic (Kleyman, 1995). In such a system, managed care providers would compete for enrollees by offering lower coverage rates than the voucher value. An elderly person would have to choose between leaving her doctors and preferred hospital, with whom she has a medical history, for an HMO or deciding not to enter a plan and keep her own providers. In not choosing managed care, the elderly person risks financial ruin if she has medical expenses beyond the voucher amount.

Converting Medicaid to a block grant also has dire consequences for the poor elderly who are disproportionately female. Medicaid would no longer be required to pay the Medicare deductibles or copayments for Part B for low-income elderly. Federal standards of eligibility, services, and quality would be weakened and the monitoring of fifty state systems would be difficult. States could also choose to eliminate coverage for high cost services such as long-term care or home care. This would be disastrous since currently about two-thirds of long-term care residents have Medicaid and the majority are female (Leadership Council of Aging Organizations, 1995).

A comprehensive caregiving policy needs to be developed for caregivers and society. Higher priority should be given to improving available choices for caregiving, ensuring a standard quality of care, and to providing financial incentives and rewards for the caregiver. Without a doubt, the elderly need wider options for available care and public financing of community care. Too often the choice is for the caregiver to lose income, have less opportunities, leave a job, or to choose expensive institutional care. Yet there has been a reduction in home-based services and support for community care in recent years. One alternative for reform would be for Medicare to pay the family to care for the elderly relative that would ensure better care at a more economical rate. The caregiver salary, however, would have to be reasonable to provide a realistic choice. Needless to say, this also raises questions about assumptions of care, the idea that women work merely for pocket money, and whether many would prefer elder care over the labor force. Another reform of a tax credit or deduction for providing home care to the elderly would be a welcomed benefit since over 80% of the home care is provided by relatives (Hess, 1985). However, Doty (1986) found that caregivers' preference in public support is for assistance and services of care over financial incentives or benefits such as tax credits or deductions.

The problem with most proposals for caregiving is the failure to address the inherent gender assumptions of care. The initial reforms must be in the family to promote gender equality and an ethic of care. Boys need to be socialized toward nurturing attitudes and to the value of providing care. The responsibilities of caregiving must be redistributed more equally between the sexes and males must assume an active role in elder care. Caregiving also needs to be perceived as a valued activity and as an investment in society. Unpaid caregiving needs to be recognized and better accommodated by the business structure of the economic system and paid caregivers need higher salaries and improved benefits.

Finally, looking toward the future there is no consensus about the prospects for older women when the Baby Boom females retire.

Some suggest that future generations of elderly women may not see much change because younger women remain in traditional jobs with low pay and because Social Security and pensions continue to be based on the male work pattern (Leonard and Loeb, 1992; Malveaux, 1993; Pifer, 1993). They see little to indicate that female Baby Boomers will not have the same situation in their later years as their mothers and grandmothers—living alone with inadequate resources. Others see positive changes for younger women that will impinge on their later years (Easterlin, MacDonald, and Macunovich, 1990; Braus, 1992). Future elderly women will be better educated and have more years of employment than the current generation of older females. Education is an important factor and closely relates to lifelong economic status. Higher education will have made future elderly women more competitive in the labor force and given them opportunities to earn better salaries and higher pension coverage. Future elderly women also will have been socialized during the feminist movement and will be more likely to push for rights and benefits. As a group, they will be more savvy and knowledgeable about finances and more concerned about gender equality. Their numbers, education, job experiences, and voices may assure greater gender justice in future public policy.

References

Allen, Jessie. (1993). The front lines. In J. Allen and A. Pifer (Eds.), *Women on the Front Lines*, pp. 1–10. Washington, DC: Urban Institute Press.

Aronson, Jane. (1992). Women's sense of responsibility for the care of old people: "But who else is going to do it?" *Gender and Society*, 6(1), 8–29.

American Association of Retired Persons (AARP). (1995) . *A Profile of Older Americans*. Washington, DC: AARP.

———. (1996). *The Social Security Book: What Every Woman Absolutely Needs to Know*. Washington, DC: AARP.

Barer, Barbara. (1994). Men and women aging differently. *International Journal of Aging and Human Development*, 38(1), 29–40.

Barr, Judith, Katrina Johnson, and Leon Warshaw. (1992). Supporting the elderly: Workforce programs for employed caregivers. *The Millbank Quarterly*, 70(3), 509–33.

Braus, Patricia. (1992). Women of a certain age. *American Demographics*, 14(12), 44–49.

Brody, Elaine, Morton Kleban, Pauline Johnsen, Christine Hoffman, and Claire Schooner. (1987). Work status and parent care: A comparison of four groups of women. *Gerontologist*, 27(2), 201–8.

Callaghan, Polly, and Heidi Hartmann. (1991). *Contingent Work: A Chart Book on Part-time and Temporary Employment*. Washington, DC: Economic Policy Institute.

Cassel, Christine, and Bernice Neugarten. (1988). A forecast of women's health and longevity-Implications for an aging America. *Western Journal of Medicine* (Women and Medicine Special Issue), 149, 712–17.

Crispell, Diane. (1995). This is your life table. *American Demographics*, 17(2), 4–6.

Doty, P. (1986). Family care: The role of public policy. *Milbank Quarterly*, 64, 34–75.

Easterlin, Richard, Christine MacDonald, and Diane Macunovich. (1990). Retirement prospects of the Baby Boom generation: A different perspective. *Gerontologist*, 30(6), 776–83.

Fahs, Marianne C. (1993). Preventive medical care: Targeting elderly women in an aging society. In J. Allen and A. Pifer (Eds.), *Women on the Front Lines*, pp. 105–31. Washington, DC: Urban Institute.

Fierst, Edith, and Nancy Duff Campbell (Eds.). (1988). *Earnings Sharing in Social Security: A Model for Reform*. Washington, DC: Center for Women Policy Studies.

Fingerhut, L. A. (1984). Changes in mortality among the elderly; United States, 1940–1978. Supplement to 1980. In *Vital and Health Statistics* (National Center for Health Statistics, U.S. Public Health Service). ser. 3, no. 22a, Department of Health and Human Services Publication No. (PHS) 82–1406a. Washington, DC: U.S. Government Printing Office. May.

Foster, Susan, and Jack Brizius. (1993). Caring too much? American women and the nation's caregiving crisis. In J. Allen and A. Pifer (Eds.), *Women on the Front Lines*, pp. 47–71. Washington, DC: The Urban Institute Press.

Gibeau, Janice L. (1989). *Adult Day Health Services as an Employee Benefit*. Washington DC National Association of Area Agencies on Aging.

Gilbert, Neil. (1994). Gender equality and Social Security. *Society*, 31(4), 27–33.

Grad, Susan. (1992). Social Security Administration, Office of Research and Statistics. Social Security Administration Publication no. 13–11871. *Income of the Population 55 or Older, 1990*. Table VI. B.2., p. 87. April.

Harpine, Cynthia, John McNeil, and Enrique Lamas. (1990). The need for personal assistance with everyday activities: Recipients and caregivers. *Current Population Reports*, ser. P–70, no. 19. U.S. Bureau of the Census. Washington, DC: U.S. Government Printing Office.

Hess, Beth. (1985). Aging policies and older women: The hidden agenda. In Alice S. Rossi (Ed.), *Gender and the Life Course*, pp. 319–31. New York: Aldine de Gruyter.

Hing, E., and B. Bloom. (1990). Long term care for the functionally dependent elderly. In *Vital and Health Statistics* (National Center for Health Statistics). ser. 13, no. 104. Hyattsville, MD: U.S. Public Health Service.

Holden, Karen. (1989). Women's economic status in old age and widowhood. In M. N. Ozawa (Ed.), *Women's Life Cycle and Economic Insecurity: Problems and Proposals*, pp. 143–69. Westport, CN: Greenwood Press.

Hudson, Robert. (1996). The changing face of aging politics. *The Gerontologist*, 36(1), 33–35.

Hurd, Michael D. (1990). Research on the elderly: Economic status, retirement and consumption and savings. *Journal of Economic Literature* (June), 565–37.

Kleyman, Paul. (1995). Budget cutters set "Policy Agenda" for older women. *Aging Today*, 16(5), 5. September/October.

Lamphere-Thorpe, Jo Ann, and Blendon, Robert. (1993). Years gained and opportunities lost: Women and healthcare in an aging society. In J. Allen and A. Pifer (Eds.), *Women on the Front Lines*, pp. 75–104. Washington, DC: Urban Institute Press.

Leader, S. (1988). Treatment of women under Medicare. In S. Sullivan and M. E. Lewin (Eds.), *The Economics and Ethics of Long Term Care and Disability*, pp. 131–44. Washington, DC: American Enterprise Institute.

Leadership Council of Aging Organizations. (1995). *Nine Different Ways: How the Budget Hurts Older Americans*. Washington, DC: Leadership Council of Aging Organizations.

Leonard, Fran, and Loeb, Laura. (1992). Heading for hardship: The future of older women in America. *USA Today Magazine*, 120(2560), 19–21. January.

Littman, Mark S. (1991). Poverty in the United States: 1990. *Current Population Reports*, ser. P–60, no. 175. U.S. Bureau of the Census. Washington, DC: U.S. Government Printing Office.

Malveaux, Julianne. (1993). Race, poverty and women's aging. In J. Allen and A. Pifer (Eds.), *Women on the Front Lines*, pp. 167–90. Washington, DC: Urban Institute Press.

Muller, Charlotte. (1983). Income support for older women. *Social Policy* (fall).

O'Grady-LeShane, Regina. (1990). Older women and poverty. *Social Work*, 35(5), 422–24.

Older Women' s League (OWL). (1989). The picture of health for midlife and older women in America. In Lois Grau (Ed.), *Women in the Later Years: Health, Social, and Cultural Perspectives*. Binghampton, NY: Harrington Park Press.

———. (1991). *Fact Sheet*. San Francisco: OWL.

Perry, D., and Robert Butler. (1988). Aim not just for a longer life, but expanded "Health Span." *Washington Post*, HE20, p. 3. 20 December.

Pifer, Alan. (1993). Meeting the challenge: Implications for policy and practice. In J. Allen and A. Pifer (Eds.), *Women on the Front Lines*, pp. 241–52. Washington, DC: Urban Institute Press.

Prescod, Margaret. (1991). *Count Women's Work: Implementing the Action Plans and Strategies of Houston and Nairobi*. Los Angeles: International Wages for Housework Campaign.

Rosenwaike, Ira, and Dolinsky, Arthur. (1987). The changing demographic determinants of the growth of the extreme aged. *Gerontologist*, 27(3), 275–80.

Rothstein, Frances R. (1994). Facts about older women: Income and poverty. *AARP Women's Initiative Fact Sheet*. Washington, DC: AARP.

Rossi, Alice S. (1985). *Gender and the Life Course*. New York: Aldine de Gruyter.

Select Committee on Aging, U.S. House of Representatives. (1988). *Exploding the Myths: Caregiving in America*. Washington, DC: U.S. Government Printing Office.

Short, Kathleen, and Nelson, Charles. (1991). Pensions: Worker coverage and retirement benefits, 1987. *Current Population Reports*, ser. P–70, no. 25. United States Bureau of the Census. Washington, DC: U.S. Government Printing Office.

Stone, Robyn, Cafferata, Gail Lee, and Sangl, Judith. (1987). Caregivers of the frail elderly: A national profile. *Gerontologist*, 27, 616–26.

Taeuber, Cynthia. (1993). U.S. Bureau of the Census, *Nursing Home Population* (Listings CPH-L-137) Table 2, p. 2. June.

———, and Allen, Jessie. (1993). Women in our aging society: The demographic outlook. In J. Allen and A. Pifer (Eds.), *Women on the Front Lines*, pp. 11-45. Washington, DC: Urban Institute Press.

Taylor, Paul. (1991). Like taking money from a baby. *Washington Post*, National Weekly Edition. 4 March, p. 31.

Turner, John, and Beller, Daniel. (1989). *Trends in Pensions*. Washington, DC: U.S. Department of Labor.

U. S. Bureau of the Census. (1991). Money income of households, families and persons in the United States: 1990. By Carmen DeNavas and Edward Welniak. *Current Population Reports*, ser. P–60, no. 174. Washington, DC: U.S. Government Printing Office.

U. S. Department of Health and Human Services. 1990. *Fast Facts and Figures and Social Security*. Washington, DC: U.S. Government Printing Office.

———. (1995). *Get a Mammogram*. Health Care Financing Administration Publication no. 10968. Washington, DC: U.S. Government Printing Office.

Zedlewski, Sheila, Barnes, Roberta, Burt, Martha, McBride, Timothy and Meyer, Jack. (1990). *The Needs of the Elderly in the 21st Century*. Washington, DC: Urban Institute Press.

Chapter 13

The Paradox of Old Age Policy
in a Changed Political Environment

TONYA M. PARROTT AND JANIE S. STECKENRIDER

Paradoxes are nothing but trouble. They violate the most
elementary principle of logic: Something cannot be two different things at once. Two contradictory interpretations cannot
both be true. A paradox is just such an impossible situation,
and political life is full of them.

—Deborah A. Stone, *Policy Paradox and Political Reason*

The new political environment is one in which paradoxes
abound, many of which have arisen out of the shifts in social values
and ideology. The preceding chapters have shown how the context
in which aging policy is made has been altered, and that the transformation—while accelerated by the events in Congress in 1994—
has been ongoing and pervasive. The paradoxes raised by the
changes are the focus of this concluding chapter, with a focus on
the policy dilemmas the changed political landscape has inspired.
This chapter ends with a summary of policy recommendations that
take into account the political environment faced by old-age policy.

Paradox #1: Individual versus Fiscal Responsibility

The new reality of aging policy is that the predominant political ideology favors self-reliance and individual and family responsibility for the needs of old age. This shift in policy is the result of

261

an intense effort to achieve deficit reduction, cost containment, and fiscal responsibility in political decision-making. While a degree of fiscal responsibility at the federal level of government is supported by Rhodebeck, Binstock, and Chen, as well by as the general public and by a growing number of academics, the contributors to this volume argue that the consequence is that families and individuals are being asked to take on more responsibility for the needs of the elderly while dually expected to share the burdens of deficit reduction. These competing policy priorities—fiscal responsibility and individual responsibility—alter the ability of individuals to care for themselves and others: while families are asked to do more, they are given less assistance and less enabling policies and resources to help them achieve this goal. The increased expectation that families should do more for the elderly makes families more vulnerable to economic constraints and places more demands on family resources. Parrott and Steckenrider point to normative assumptions about family life and gender roles to explain these contradictory social policy values while Binstock, Torres-Gil, and Day point to changes in the political players and the political party in power as additional explanations.

In part, the focus on scaling back spending on Medicare and Medicaid as a way to cut government costs and to find budget "savings" is an inevitable outcome of fiscal responsibility; as Binstock suggests, Medicare is a likely target for deficit reduction because it is such a large part of the federal budget outlays and it is under federal control (so it can be tampered with). The implication of fiscal responsibility in the area of health care policy is that there will be less government assistance to elders for their health care needs and there will be a higher expectation that seniors cover the increasing out-of-pocket expenses that will follow, including the growing cost of long-term care. Moreover, Steckenrider and Villa demonstrate that the long-term and gender- and minority-based health care needs of the older population are not well-served by current policy. Instead of trying innovative or alternative mechanisms to deal with the changing needs of the older population itself, the primary policy action has been to tinker with the health care system we have, while slicing away at the benefits that are offered. In short, these policies have asked the elderly to cover more of their own health care expenses while offering scaled back health care coverage that is inadequate for a large portion of the older population.

Binstock and Rhodebeck indicate that just as Medicare changes seem inevitable if the government is to achieve deficit reduction, demographic realism cannot be avoided either. The numbers of the elderly will continue to grow, and despite whatever changes occur in health care financing, the costs of health care will rise and the projected trust fund problems will not vanish because the sheer quantity of those in need among the ranks of the elderly will continue to grow as the Baby Boomers age and as frail elders with chronic conditions live longer. As Chen shows, this means there will be a greater need for more alternative forms of income security in old age, over and above whatever assistance will be available through the public pension system, to be able to afford health care costs and the financing of daily needs over a longer period of time. Chen offers alternatives to the current model of income security that take into account the changes within the older population, the need for greater fiscal responsibility on the part of government, and the increasing demands that are being placed on individuals and families to plan for their own long-term economic security and needs in old age. He suggests redesigning the Social Security system to reflect part-time work patterns among semiretired seniors in combination with a rise in the normal retirement age, based on the life expectancy of tomorrow's elderly cohorts.

Liebig, Parrott, Villa, and Steckenrider argue that there will be considerable inequality in the way that the goal of fiscal responsibility is operationalized, particularly in the differential impact it will have on subgroups of the older population. Inaccurate, outdated, or biased assumptions about family, women's roles and abilities, and minority needs and preferences exist across policy domains. For example, Liebig shows that elderly white females, Hispanics, and African-Americans have inadequate rental housing and are poorer than other subgroups of the elderly. Moreover, Liebig shows that for many poor or minority elderly, their housing expenses are higher than their health care costs, especially among female renters aged 75 and older. Villa and Steckenrider echo these disparities. Villa shows that within the minority elderly population limited work opportunities and benefit reductions in Social Security and Medicare lead to greater income disparity and more reliance on public assistance programs in old age compared to the situation for nonminorities. Older females, as Steckenrider demonstrates, are often on the edge of poverty because they are penalized for being unpaid homemakers and caregivers, remain concentrated in lower-paying jobs, and are assumed to be the primary caregivers for children and elders. These assumptions about family roles and duties, Steckenrider and Parrott argue, are institutionalized into our value system and into our public policies. These authors characterize current policies for our aging society as being based on a male, white non-Hispanic, traditional family model of health, mortality, work life, and caregiving responsibility. As a result, the burden of financing more years of life with chronic conditions, potentially expensive nursing home care, inadequate housing arrangements, and caregiving responsibilities falls disproportionately on women and minorities.

While perhaps these assumptions were appropriate for an aging population in earlier times, today's population aging is a largely female, and increasingly minority, experience. Data presented within this volume indisputably identify those most in need of assistance—the most vulnerable of the elderly—as aged 75 and older individuals who are female, minority, poor, uneducated, with disrupted work histories, single or widowed, renters, and in HMOs or other managed care cost containment systems of health care delivery. Change is needed, but the approaches offered by the various authors reflect the paradox of more responsibility being placed on individuals and families as a result of more attention to fiscal responsibility. Possibly the greatest individual responsibility falls on those elderly who are the least prepared for it: the poor and near-poor, minorities, and older women living alone.

Paradox #2: Doing More With Less

Fernando Torres-Gil, former Assistant Secretary of Aging, succinctly stated that the major dilemma for old-age policy is to figure out how to do more for those in need with fewer federal resources and with the increased expectation for them to take on more personal responsibility. Increased burdens on the family will produce strains on other social institutions (e.g., the workplace, and the formal support system). Families increasingly will need to turn to formal, community-based assistance to meet eldercare demands, but long-term, community-based social support and affordable assisted housing do not appear to be forthcoming.

For example, Binstock sees the national focus on limiting Medicaid expenses (the major public funding option for long-term care) as further limiting any future expenditures on long-term care, despite the increased need for it by the aging population. Moreover, as states look for ways to limit the cost of Medicaid, Binstock discloses that some have considered discontinuing all community-based long-term care financing. Liebig confirms that federal rescissions in budgets for innovative housing and social service linkages limit the potential for expanding this type of assistance in housing settings. Thus, while community-based long-term care options are the most needed policy innovations, they are the least likely to emerge. According to Binstock, nursing homes will continue to get more of the attention and dollars of state governments than will more public home-care options because the physical structures already exist and because "nursing home residents have nowhere else to go." Liebig argues that pressures for developers to make a profit combined with a less active federal government role in providing affordable housing options will mean more alternatives for the well-off elderly and even greater inequality and limited choices for low-income elders. The net result is that community-based efforts to meet increased formal care needs will amount to attempts at providing more of these kinds of services with fewer resources.

But, as states have more power over programs for the elderly, they will also become more financially strapped. Federal block grant amounts to states, for example, may be lower than the previous matching amounts states were receiving with Medicaid. And, despite the shift in power over many programs from the federal government to the states and municipalities, Day, Binstock, and Liebig suggest that there will not be much interest group activity at the lower levels of government to lobby for how the resources are allocated. Even if there were more interest group mobilization at the lower levels, it is likely to perpetuate current practices among groups (e.g., a narrow focus, little coalition-building, and a lack of representation for the poor elderly) which would lead to greater disparity in the allocation of public dollars. Equally important, Rhodebeck shows that state- and local-level intergenerational conflicts may emerge over budgetary priorities. Who has the power to influence policymakers—interest groups and individuals alike—will continue to be a crucial predictor of how old-age policy is made. Day suggests that the groups influencing current policymakers have changed. She points to the emergence of the Seniors Coalition, the United Seniors Association (USA), and the 60/Plus Association as new age-related interest groups that sprung up in the mid-1990s, and explains that these new groups fall on the more conservative end of the policy priority continuum. Notably, these are groups that support the idea of seniors and families doing more for themselves with less government assistance. Meanwhile, Binstock notes that the American Association of Retired Persons (AARP), the largest age-based interest group, is unlikely to take too political of a stance on issues such as changes in Medicare or Social Security because it must be concerned with protecting its nonpartisan claims and retaining its members.

Technological advances in political participation may actually open more doors for senior participation in the political system to influence policy decisions about how to "do more with less" at all levels of government. If the interpretations of data and the forecasts offered by Day, Rhodebeck, MacManus, and Tenpas are correct, then two things can be assumed: (1) the participation rates of seniors will remain strong or even rise as the numbers of seniors increase, as a more educated and politically active cohort of Baby Boomers age, as new technologies make it easier for seniors to participate in the political process, and as politicians go to where the seniors are (e.g., senior centers, and retirement communities) to solicit their votes; and (2) in addition to a focus on the cost of programs, when politicians are faced with votes related to budgetary priorities for different age groups they will continue to consider the preferences of the elderly who vote in their districts or states. Many intergenerational equity advocates are concerned that seniors will support "doing more with less" by voting to cut funding for local school districts. In general, Rhodebeck concludes, the elderly can be expected to support education policy at the local level, although not necessarily as strongly as other age groups. Furthermore, Parrott's chapter suggests that changes in family life such as grandparents having relationships with grandchildren and grandparents actually raising grandchildren will make seniors feel more connected to, and invested in, intergenerational issues. This may moderate any potential local level age-group tensions over decisions about doing more with less. Thus, policy decisions about resource allocations come down to who votes and how they vote: seniors vote more, although their vote preferences reflect social class, political ideology, and individual and cohort experiences.

The last part of the paradox of "doing more with less" is that those senior citizens most in need among the elderly are the least likely to receive policy attention. Day and Liebig remind us that interest groups tend to underrepresent the poor in any policy domain, and they suggest that the current policy trends toward greater personal responsibility, less federal government involvement in daily life, and reduced funding levels in general, suggest no improvement in this situation. Villa argues that the problem with government policies placing more responsibility on individuals and families is that there is no equality of opportunity for all and that the social system places barriers in the way of minorities that are "beyond their control" while holding them to the same standard of responsibility as those elders who are more privileged. Diverse, broad-based coalitions that might bring together groups representing cross-generational, cross-class, and multicultural concerns are not given much hope in Day's view, while Torres-Gil predicts there will be more of an intergenerational focus on policy, with decision-makers giving greater emphasis and priority to policies that serve more than one group.

Paradox #3: Status Quo or Change?

Within the context of a changed political environment, policy priorities fall into two competing agendas: (1) maintaining the status quo and continuing the course of policy action that has been followed in the past (e.g., continuing to support current old-age policies so that the elderly—as an eligibility group—are able to retain as many resources and benefits as possible); or (2) using the changed political environment as a time to assess existing policies and how successful they are in achieving policy goals in contrast to pilot programs and experimental approaches that are less costly or controlled locally rather than federally (e.g., terminating unsuccessful or flawed old-age policies and trying new ones).

Blancato and Lindberg suggest that the goal of the aging policy community should be reaffirming support for current programs (status quo). Torres-Gil recommends that the Older Americans Act (OAA) be given more support, especially because of the role that it could play in delivering more community-based services to those families and individuals in need (status quo). Many authors, however, call for a reassessment of current policies to make them more in line with the current and future older population's needs, particularly when it comes to out-of-pocket health care expenses, chronic health conditions, long-term and community-based care needs, economic insecurity for older minorities and women, and shifts in family structure and caregiving.

Liebig recommends an evaluation of the policy choices that have been made in housing and a reconsideration of where the few remaining federal resources are allocated (change). Chen and Steckenrider advocate new designs for the financing and benefit structure of Social Security (change). Binstock calls for new approaches to health care that link acute care with long-term care (change), while Villa is looking for greater overall access to the health care system (change). Parrott raises the issue of why some workplace and caregiving policies appear underutilized or ineffective (change), while Steckenrider argues that caregiving is a second shift for older women— much like child care is for younger women— and thus it must be valued socially and economically (change). In various ways, each author argues that existing old age policies are not the policies that are needed because changes in the older population itself and in family structure have taken place. In short, a challenge is made to the status quo and to its accompanying incremental approach to policy-making for the elderly in the new political environment.

A laundry list of policy proposals are offered by the contributors to this volume: (1) better access to health care, a public long-term care policy, and more preventive health care options for women; (2) affordable supportive housing, and more support and funding for OAA programs; (3) changes in Social Security benefit calculations to reflect longer life expectancies, gendered work histories, and caregiving roles, and a way to finance caregiving assistance; (4) better educational and occupational opportunities for minorities so that they are prepared—financially and physically—for old age, and more recognition and elimination of the differential effects of economic policies and health policies on the subpopulations of the elderly most in need. Support for these proposals and the likelihood that any of them will be acted upon will be tempered by the new political environment and by the competing approaches of sustaining the status quo or pursuing policy changes.

Blancato and Lindberg argue that because of the new political environment, agenda setting during the 1995 White House Conference on Aging (WHCoA) was not revolutionary despite the revolutionary rhetoric in Washington, DC, at the time the conference took place. Rather, the 1995 WHCoA was a pragmatic process based on a formula: (1) incremental changes are the best and most successful in times of government retrenchment; (2) preserving existing programs is primary; and (3) changes can be considered only if they are not costly, can actually save money, or can keep expenses at the same level but can deliver service or assistance more effectively. Their proposed policy-making approach is inherently paradoxical— incremental changes are favored over dramatic, broad-based changes while, at the same time, change is desirable if it can be shown to save the government money. Saving money would require doing away with some of the current policies in favor of more innovative, experimental models or dramatically revamping the benefit structure and financing of some programs. Thus, Blancato and Lindberg illustrate the paradoxical nature of public policy-making.

Torres-Gil, Binstock, Blancato, and Lindberg argue that while publicly financed long-term care is clearly the "missing link" in health care policy for an aging society, the political climate dictates that this subject is virtually off-limits. Binstock says that while private long-term care financing options exist, they are inaccessible and unaffordable for most seniors and their families and the practice of asset sheltering is an unfair way to finance long-term care because it is an informal yet pervasive policy approach that does not help those most in need and it places greater burden on state budgets. Thus, instead of fostering savings, some implicit policy choices can lead to greater government costs in the extreme and greater social inequities in the most mundane of circumstances.

Given that the acute health care system for the aged is in financial trouble, Binstock raises the issue of how it will be possible to finance long-term care, especially when the political mood in federal politics is antigovernment expansion. Rhodebeck suggests that entitlement programs such as Social Security cannot be left off-limits by any politician who is serious about deficit reduction. Because politicians look at the reelection consequences of their votes, however, it is unlikely that real policy change will take place or that there will be any dramatic change in the policy choices that have already been made. This may be true despite the acknowledgment that policy change is the only real way to control the deficit.

Recommendations

In spite of the paradoxical nature of the changed political environment, with its increased focus on social values and policy choices, several recommendations from contributors are possible and in concert with the new context of policy-making for an aging society.

The first paradox requires a balance between individual and fiscal responsibility. This will mean more and better targeting of resources in all areas, including more cost-sharing and private-market alternatives. Large federal programs are no longer options for dealing with the problems of old age. By definition, this translates to less universalism in benefit eligibility and access and more means-testing. In targeting efforts, policymakers and program administrators must focus on the *intragenerational* diversity of the older population now and in the future, identifying those most in need within these subgroups. In this way, the inequity that can result from fiscal responsibility will not fall too heavily on those who are the least prepared to handle it. Decisions about targeting resources should involve an open discussion of public value preferences. Who should public assistance help most—middle-class families dealing with long-term care expenses or low-income elders in poverty and poor health? Torres-Gil, from his unique perspective, argues that for any proposal to be successful it will have to have embedded within it the values of self-reliance and individual responsibility. How will these values get operationalized in aging policy? Probably through more family responsibility initiatives, more cost-sharing, and less federal public assistance options.

The second paradox requires governments and families to do more for the elderly with fewer federal resources. To that end, there will need to be more flexibility in policy boundaries and government rules regarding eligibility determinations for benefits and the financing and implementation of programs. More public-private efforts will be necessary both in terms of program choices and mechanisms for financing them. Given that state and local governments will have more control of programs for the elderly, there will need to be room for adaptation and experimentation in order to find new ways to provide community-based alternatives for linking long-term and acute care, supportive services and housing, family caregiving needs and other work and family demands, minority needs in programs offered and ability to access these programs, and public and private savings approaches for old age. While state initiatives are identified as crucial by numerous authors, the promise for realizing this may not be encouraging because states are strapped for funds and will increasingly face additional fiscal pressures and competing needy groups as changes to the social safety net are carried out (e.g., the elimination of Aid to Families with Dependent Children). In short, doing more with less will necessitate more public-private and private alternatives to the problems of old age.

The third policy paradox is whether to support the status quo in aging policy or to favor changing policies—reassessing their value in today's political environment or reallocating the resources elsewhere. To guide decision-making in this area, grass roots interest groups and coalitions are needed and should be fostered at the state and local levels of government. New strategies must be developed to advocate for the intergenerational needs of an aging society because the legitimacy of groups depends not only on who is in power in government but also on the competing demands of other organized interests and how they frame the issues. A more *intergenerational* focus will need to pervade proposals and options for the status quo or to change in order to garner cross-age-group support for the allocation of state and local moneys and so that whatever the policy outcome—status quo or change—it is perceived as a fair and equitable solution. The crucial policy choice for the future is whether old-age programs will even remain a priority. This volume suggests that intergenerational proposals may receive more resources in the years to come.

Conclusions

While certainly not a picture of expansion and growth, the outlook for old-age programs is not entirely one of loss. The 1995 White House Conference on Aging acted to reaffirm support for, and commitment to, the major programs serving the elderly: Social Security, Medicare, Medicaid, and the Older Americans Act. Beyond just confirming allegiance to the programs, the fight to keep them intact speaks to the success that many of these programs have had in improving the conditions of old age.

However, in periods of cultural change such as now where there is a shift in the prevailing ideas and values about government versus personal responsibility for the condition and well-being of individuals, policymakers and program planners are forced to find new and innovative ways to run programs and to meet needs. Times of intense social scrutiny offer opportunities to discontinue programs that are not working and to start again. Thus, this may be the very time to assess the value of various experimental programs as alternatives to the programs we so freely criticize (e.g., Social Security and problems with its benefit distributions) but so dearly try to hold on to when their livelihood is threatened (e.g., reductions in the growth in Medicare spending). New ideas bring new approaches to problem-solving and, in the long-run, may actually leave us with better-operating state- and local-level programs and new public-private options. There will definitely be growing pains that are felt by many as the policy environment continues to change, but perhaps the pains will not be as bad as some have predicted if we are willing to adapt, be innovative, and better-skilled at targeting those who stand to benefit the most from our policy interventions.

References

Stone, Deborah A. (1988). *Policy Paradox and Political Reason*. New York: Harper Collins.

About the Editors

Janie S. Steckenrider, Ph.D., is associate professor of political science at Loyola Marymount University in Los Angeles, California. Her research focuses on seniors' political attitudes and behavior, elderly health issues, and gender politics. She has published articles in the *Encyclopedia of Aging, the Journal of Women and Politics, the Southwest Journal on Aging, the Policy Studies Journal,* and *the American Journal of Alzheimer's Care and Research*. She has served on the boards of directors of a hospital, a skilled nursing facility, an Alzheimer's disease research foundation, and a municipal senior citizens commission.

Tonya M. Parrott, Ph.D., is assistant professor of sociology and gerontology at Quinnipiac College in Hamden, Connecticut. She earned her B.A. in sociology from UCLA and her Ph.D. in gerontology and public policy from the University of Southern California. A National Institute of Aging Predoctoral Research Fellow for four years, she was only the fourth person in the country to earn a doctorate in gerontology. Her research interests include aging and the family, intergenerational relations, and the relationship between social values and policy choices for an aging society. She has coauthored articles in the *Journal of Marriage and the Family, The Gerontologist*, the *Journal of Gerontology: Social Sciences*, and *Research on Aging*.

About the Contributors

Robert H. Binstock, Ph.D., is professor of aging, health, and society, at Case Western Reserve University. A former president of the Gerontological Society of America (1975–76), he has served as director of a White House Task Force on Older Americans for President Lyndon B. Johnson, and as chairman and member of a number of advisory panels to the federal, state and local governments; and foundations. He presently chairs the Gerontological Health Section of the American Public Health Association. He has published some 150 articles and book chapters dealing with politics and policies on aging. Among his 19 authored and edited books are four editions of the *Handbook of Aging and the Social Sciences* (the most recent, coedited with Linda K. George).

Robert B. Blancato has been involved in national aging policy for more than 20 years, including 15 years of service in Congress, primarily as staff director of the House Select Committee on Aging, Subcommittee on Human Services. He was appointed by President Clinton to serve as the executive director of the 1995 White House Conference on Aging. He now provides public and government relations consulting in the firm of Matz, Shea, and Blancato.

Yung-Ping Chen, Ph.D., holds the Frank J. Manning Eminent Scholar's Chair in Gerontology at the University of Massachusetts, Boston. A delegate to the 1971, 1981, and 1995 White House conferences on aging, he also served on the Panel of Actuaries and Economists of the 1979 Advisory Council of Social Security. A fellow in the Gerontological Society of America, he served as 1992–93 chair of the Economics of Aging Formal Interest Group and editor of its newsletter (1988–93). He is a founding member of the National Academy of Social Insurance and was its visiting scholar in 1989.

Christine L. Day, Ph.D., is associate professor of political science at the University of New Orleans. She is the author of *What Older Americans Think: Interest Groups and Aging Policy* and has published articles on interest groups, public opinion, and public policy, including articles on aging policy in the *Journal of Politics* and *Research on Aging*.

Phoebe S. Liebig, Ph.D., is associate professor of gerontology and public administration at the Andrus Gerontology Center, University of Southern California. She conducts research on intergovernmental issues and state-level policy in housing, disability, and long-term care. A former senior policy analyst with the Public Policy Institute of the American Association of Retired Persons, she has published articles in the *Journal of Aging and Social Policy* and *Publius: The Journal of Federalism*. Recent writings include *Housing Frail Elders: International Policies, Perspectives, and Prospects*, coedited with Jon Pynoos, and "The Effects of Federalism on

Policies for Care of the Aged in Canada and the United States" in
the *Journal of Aging and Social Policy*.

Brian W. Lindberg is the executive director of the Consumer
Coalition for Quality Health Care, which advocates for consumer
information, appeals rights, consumer advocate programs, and a
system of independent quality oversight. He worked in Congress
for ten years, including service as staff director of a House Select
Committee on Aging subcommittee and on the Senate Special Committee on Aging.

Susan A. MacManus, Ph.D., is professor of public administration and political science at the University of South Florida,
Tampa. She is president of the Urban Politics Section of the American Political Science Association. She sits on the editorial boards of
several major policy and public administration journals and has
published works on public policy, budgeting and finance, intergovernmental fiscal relations, and women and minorities in numerous
journals, including the *Journal of Politics*, *Public Administration
Review*, the *Policy Studies Journal*, the *American Journal of Political Science*, and *Urban Affairs Quarterly*. One of her three books
published in the past few years is *Young v. Old: Generational Combat in the 21st Century*. She served on the Florida Governor's Council of Economic Advisors and was a Fulbright Research Scholar at
Yonsei University, Seoul, Korea (1989).

Laurie A. Rhodebeck, Ph.D., is assistant professor of political science at the State University of New York, Buffalo. Her research focuses on public opinion and voting behavior in American
politics. She recently published an article, "The Politics of Greed?
Political Preferences Among the Elderly," in the *Journal of Politics*
and is currently working on a project that examines how social and
political contexts shape public opinion about age policy.

Kathryn Dunn Tenpas, Ph.D., is assistant professor at the
University of South Florida. Her research has been published in
Presidential Studies Quarterly, *Political Science Quarterly*, and the
Journal of Law and Politics. She is completing a book entitled,
*Presidents as Candidates: Inside the White House for the Presiden-
tial Campaign*.

Fernando M. Torres-Gil, Ph.D., is professor in the School of
Public Policy and Social Research at the University of California,
Los Angeles, with joint appointments in the Department of Social
Welfare and the Department of Policy Studies. He previously served
as the first assistant secretary for aging in the Department of Health
and Human Services (1993–96). He was charged with overseeing

aging policy within the department as well as throughout the federal government, providing leadership for the Administration on Aging, and serving as the focal point for assuring that a system of aging services is provided at the state and local levels. He was president of the American Society on Aging (1990–92), and has served in a variety of governmental positions, including staff director for the U.S. House of Representatives Select Committee on Aging (1985–87), special assistant to then-secretary of health and human services, Patricia Roberts Harris, and special assistant to Joseph Califano, secretary of health, education, and welfare (1978-79). He was appointed by President Jimmy Carter to the Federal Council on Aging in 1978 and in 1990–92 he served as a member of the Social Security Administration's Supplemental Security Income Modernization Task Force.

Valentine M. Villa, Ph.D., is Assistant Professor in the School of Public Policy and Social Research at the University of California, Los Angeles. Her research interest is in the health status of minority populations, particularly investigation of the determinants of health status. Her publications include examinations of the determinants of disease and functioning among Korean, African-American, and Hispanic elders. She currently teaches aging policy, research methods in aging, and organizational and community theory.

Author Index

Subject Index